THE HUMAN
GENOME PROJECT
AND THE FUTURE
OF HEALTH CARE

Medical Ethics Series
David H. Smith and Robert M. Veatch, Editors

The Human Genome Project and the Future of Health Care

edited by Thomas H. Murray, Mark A. Rothstein, and Robert F. Murray, Jr.

INDIANA UNIVERSITY PRESS

Bloomington and Indianapolis

The paper used in this publication
meets the minimum requirements of American National Standard
for Information Sciences—Permanence of Paper
for Printed Library Materials,
ANSI Z39.48-1984.

Manufactured in the United States of America

Library of Congress Cataloging-in-Publication Data

The Human Genome Project and the future of health care / edited by
Thomas H. Murray, Mark A. Rothstein, and Robert F. Murray, Jr.
p.   cm. — (Medical ethics series)
Includes index.
ISBN 0-253-33213-3 (cl : alk. paper)
1. Human Genome Project—Social aspects.   2. Human Genome Project—
Moral and ethical aspects.   I. Murray, Thomas H. (Thomas Harold),
date.   II. Rothstein, Mark A.   III. Murray, Robert F.
IV. Series.
QH445.2.H87   1996
174′.2–dc20   96-1718

2 3 4 5   01 00 99 98 97

Contents

Introduction:
The Human Genome Project
and the Future of Health Care

Thomas H. Murray

The contributions to this volume share a thesis: that the Human Genome Project, in combination with other forces, will reshape health care in the United States. To put it more fully, if the general problem of access to health care is the question, "Who will offer what to whom at whose expense?" the HGP will substantially alter the Who, the What, and the To Whom, and may also affect the At Whose Expense? Each of these questions is linked to access and each has important ethical dimensions.

The Who doing the offering are health professionals, predominantly physician-geneticists and non-physician genetic counselors. That may change dramatically in the future as the burden of interpreting genetic information falls increasingly heavily on primary-care physicians not trained as geneticists and on other health professionals such as nurse-practitioners who may come to be seen as a more cost-effective way of providing primary-care services (Jonsen, chapter 1). What must be done to assure that these professionals are equipped to be skillful interpreters of genetic information (Riccardi, chapter 2)? The What is likely to expand greatly as a broad variety of genetic services and genetic information enter both primary and specialty care. Some of these will be extensions of familiar services, though they may bring their own problems—a vastly increased menu of possible choices for prenatal diagnosis. Others will be technical novelties, but may fit readily into available paradigms for assimilating expensive new technologies—using recombinant DNA techniques to treat cancer, for example (Polvino and Anderson, chapter 3). In their costs, risks, and potential benefits such adaptations of gene therapy may resemble closely other therapeutic innovations for cancer treatment, such as new drugs or bone marrow transplantation. The To Whom lies at the heart of justice. Who shall benefit from these new genetic technologies (Nickens, chapter 4; Bobinski, chapter 5; Mehlman, chapter 6)? Will their high cost limit access to those with gold-plated private health insurance? Will genetic prediction of risk of disease be used to exclude from health care coverage those most likely to need it (Stone, chapter 7; Asch, chapter 8)? At Whose Expense also touches on justice: How should the financial burden of illness be distributed? Together with the previous question, the issue of financing health care compels us to ask what the social institution of health insurance is intended to accomplish, and whether we should view genetic and other diseases as a matter of one's personal fate, or as a shared community responsibility (Daniels, chapter 9).

What are the most significant implications of the Human Genome Project for access to health care for clinicians (R. F. Murray, chapter 10), for ethics (T. H. Murray, chapter 11), and for public policy (Rothstein, chapter 12)?

Albert R. Jonsen begins our exploration of the Human Genome Project's impact on the future of health care by extending the mapping analogy, which has been so influential in the project, to the future of the patient-physician relationship. He describes four important features of that relationship likely to be affected by the Genome Project. First will be a drawing of the Future into the Present as the prospect of future disease, based on genetic risks or predispositions, becomes an increasingly important part of health care. Second is a movement from Possibility to Actuality in what Jonsen calls "ordinary life psychology." Rather than the risks of future disease being seen as outside oneself and probabilistic, Jonsen argues that they will come to be seen as "written in each person's genome, an indelible part of the self." The third shift will be from a *Scientia Activa* to a *Scientia Contemplativa*, a somewhat ironic return to medicine's past, when it could offer diagnosis and prognosis but do little to alter the course of disease, at least until the discoveries of genomic science bear therapeutic fruit. Fourth comes an enlarging of the relationship from the patient-physician Duality to the Multitude of persons interested in and possibly affected by genetic information, including biological relatives, and providing increasing opportunities for screening large populations for genetic risks. Jonsen observes that the reductionism that seems to go hand-in-glove with modern medicine may be exacerbated by the genome's impact if physicians focus on genes and molecules rather than the person in whom those genes and molecules reside. But he also holds out hope that the four shifts he identifies may rescue medicine from reductionism.

Given the vast increase in the amount of genetic information likely to come in the near future, the fact that only about 1,000 genetics professionals—M.D. geneticists and genetic counselors—are currently available in the United States is alarming. One promising strategy is to educate clinicians about genetics. Vincent M. Riccardi's chapter is addressed to clinicians, educators, and policy makers. Riccardi is concerned with enhancing "genetic literacy" among the public broadly, but especially among clinicians, who, he notes, are increasingly being asked to act as managers and to take financial considerations into account in their management of patients. As genetics in clinical practice is transformed from the esoteric to the mundane, clinicians will have to become skilled interpreters of genetic information. Reviewing new developments in diagnosis and treatment, Riccardi argues that the diagnosis and treatment of genetic disease can no longer be left to geneticists. Finally, he describes the techniques and resources available for educating clinicians about genetics.

As important as increased genetic diagnosis and prediction are, much of the hope for the Genome Project rests on the possibility of new therapies, including most notably human gene therapy. William J. Polvino and W. French Anderson conduct research on gene therapy. In their chapter they provide a brief history of the technology and an equally brief description of its results thus far. With this as background, they describe the surprising—and growing—array of possible uses. Gene therapy, initially conceived as a possible treatment for very rare, single-gene disorders, is now touted for its potential therapeutic value against cancer, heart disease, and even AIDS. They describe the many barriers—regulatory, technological, and financial—that gene therapy will have to surmount before it can benefit large numbers of people.

If history is any guide, the benefits—and the burdens—of the Genome Project will not fall evenly on all groups. Herbert Nickens warns that the interval in which we will know a great deal about the location and sequence of genes, but much less about their significance, will be a kind of Rorschach test for society, and "a perilous time" for minorities. With human genetics as the preeminent "science of inequality," the Genome Project will provide further specification of the biological differences between persons. Nickens is concerned about how that information will be used in a nation with "a long and disturbing history of drawing sharp distinctions among our citizens on the basis of race and ethnicity" as well as "a long tradition of belief in biological determinism." Nickens reviews briefly some of the episodes that have helped to fuel suspicion among minorities that genetic information may not be used to their benefit. He describes the potential for an explosive mixture of race and genetics by offering an illuminating contrast of the responses to cystic fibrosis, sickle-cell anemia, and low birthweight. He concludes his chapter by addressing concerns about non-medical uses of genetic information and discrimination against minorities.

To the extent that reproductive decisions are affected by the Genome Project, the impact is likely to fall disproportionately on women. Mary Anne Bobinski considers the implications of genomic science for reproductive health. As prenatal genetic testing and screening yields more information for more women, questions will arise about the voluntariness of such testing, and about access to genetic services. Should eugenic pressures increase, especially pressure not to have children with genetic conditions that are expensive to care for, women may find themselves pushed to undergo testing, and perhaps into not continuing pregnancies when fetuses are identified with such conditions.

A third group of persons who might receive less than their share of the health care benefits of the Genome Project are those whose health care coverage comes from federal programs like Medicare and Medicaid. Maxwell J. Mehlman analyzes how such entitlement programs regulate access to other health care technologies as a guide to how they are likely to control access to genome-related technologies. He notes that more than one-quarter of all health care benefits in the United States are paid for by either Medicare or Medicaid, and that these two programs serve principally two groups: those who cannot afford their own health care, and those who society has decided should not have to pay for themselves—the affluent elderly. Mehlman argues that public programs of health care coverage will experience increasing pressures to contain cost. To the extent that genome-inspired health care technologies, especially expensive ones such as gene therapy, increase cost, government programs will have to rely on increasing copayments, restricting what services are covered, or constraining availability. He does not believe that government programs will succeed in limiting eligibility for coverage. Mehlman foresees the possibility that effective—but costly— genetic technologies will be available only to those with expensive private insurance or sufficient wealth to purchase them independently. The less affluent, including most people covered under government programs, will have to rely on other methods; in a chilling passage, Mehlman describes abortion as "the poor person's gene therapy." He worries about a sharp division of the country into those who can afford genetic therapies, and perhaps genetic enhancements as well, and those who cannot.

Deborah A. Stone examines the implications of the Genome Project for access to health insurance. She argues that information about genetic risks will exacerbate a trend which has seen insurers try ever harder to selectively insure those likely to remain relatively healthy, leaving those most at risk of illness at the mercy of public programs, just those buffeted by the forces identified by Mehlman. Stone looks very carefully at the sources of health-risk-related information that insurers exploit, from medical records to "inspection reports" from agencies that interview friends, neighbors, and co-workers. She analyzes the conception of fairness that underlies the practice of insurance underwriting—linking access and cost of coverage to the likelihood of filing a claim. She concludes with a pessimistic exploration of the possibilities for restricting insurers' access to genetic information, and with a hope that the Genome Project might spur us to reexamine our provisions for access to health care coverage in the United States.

Nearly two-thirds of Americans under age 65 who have health insurance get it through an employer-provided policy. Adrienne Asch examines the implications of the Genome Project for employment, and for the access to health insurance that flows from employment. Asch argues that how we deal with genetics is inextricably entwined with how we deal with disabilities, whatever their etiology. She shows that the Americans with Disabilities Act (ADA), though a great advance, does not protect people with disabilities or their family members from a number of possible problems related to employment, ranging from covert discrimination, to inadequate coverage of health care costs, to being trapped in a job because changing jobs could lead to lapses or complete loss of needed health care coverage. Asch also explores the link between work and health, arguing that even if we sever the link between employment and health care coverage, having useful work is important to both physical and mental health.

Norman Daniels takes on three philosophical questions crucial for mediating the impact of the Human Genome Project on access to health care. First, he examines the implications of using genetic information to predict such things as the likelihood of extended survival for transplant recipients. If genetic information suggests that, of two candidates for a heart transplant, one has a gene indicating a risk for another disease five, ten, or twenty years hence, while the other has no comparable risks, should the transplant go to the individual without the added risk? As Daniels frames the question, "What weight should we give to assuring 'best outcomes' rather than giving people 'equal chance at an important benefit'?" He then picks up a theme introduced by Stone—whether it is fair to deny access to health insurance coverage on the grounds that an individual is at increased risk for disease. Daniels puts it this way: "What are our moral obligations to share these risks despite improved information about them?" Finally, he tackles one of the knottiest problems in health care, one likely to be exacerbated as we gain the capacity to manipulate our physiology and anatomy—the distinction between therapy and enhancement. Daniels asks: "Can we defend the distinction between medical technologies that treat and those that enhance in the face of new genetic information that allows us to pinpoint the genetic contributors to traits we want to alter?"

The editors of this volume contribute the last three chapters. Robert F. Murray, Jr., summarizes the implications of the Human Genome Project for clinical practice, with special attention to recent changes in the health care system. Thomas H. Murray considers two critical ethical issues: the problem of justice in access to health care, and the distinction between therapy and enhancement. Finally, Mark A. Rothstein surveys the key policy issues mediating the impact of the Human Genome Project on health care access. He pays explicit attention to problems arising from public financing of health care, in the realm of reproductive autonomy, and the role of employers. He concludes his chapter, and this volume, with suggestions for a legislative and policy agenda.

THE HUMAN
GENOME PROJECT
AND THE FUTURE
OF HEALTH CARE

One

The Impact of Mapping the Human Genome on the Patient-Physician Relationship

Albert R. Jonsen

The gradual discovery of the loci of the 100,000 genes in the human genome will be like the European discovery of unknown lands. Following 1492, many changes, some good, some evil, affected human life and culture. The mapping of the genome will similarly change science and medicine in many ways. Among the many changes, it will require the redrawing of the lines that mark the present boundaries of the relationship between physicians and their patients, just as maps had to be redrawn during the Age of Exploration. By the middle of the twenty-first century, the genomic physician and the genomic patient will look upon each other from quite different standpoints than they do today. Naturally, like territorial boundaries in remote areas, the boundaries of the patient-physician relationship as it has existed and as it will exist in the genomic era will often overlap. Some territories will remain in the old domain; many of the new features will resemble the old. Still, it is likely that the map of the relationship will become a new one as the scientific work of mapping the genome proceeds. This chapter, then, will sketch the broad outlines of that future map.

The Mapping Metaphor

The project to map the human genome began in the late 1980s and its progress is described in other chapters in this book. While the scientific

1

progress has been rapid and remarkable in the development of methods for mapping and even in the identification of many genes, only a tiny fragment of the genome has yet been mapped and only a few human diseases have been linked to that map. This chapter depicts the future relationships between physicians and patients that may come into being once a fully realized genome map is drawn. Any depiction of an as-yet unrealized future will be rather like the fanciful creations of those medieval cartographers who drew maps of places that no one had ever seen. Thus, any implications for the relationship between patient and physician are speculative and probable. This speculative and probable topic can be rendered more concrete and visible through a metaphor: the metaphor of map making. This is, of course, the master metaphor for the entire scientific enterprise known loosely as "The Genome Project." Many authors have utilized the metaphor in an extended sense. For example, James Watson and Norton Zinder vividly employed the metaphor in a letter to the *New York Times*: "Like the system of state highways spanning our country, the map of the human genome will be completed stretch by stretch."[1]

The metaphor, in its specific application to the scientific work of creating linkage maps and physical maps, or in its more extended sense of describing the scope and design of the project, is of course an inexact analogy. Mapmaking, properly speaking, involves using pen and paper to draw squiggly lines within Mercator projections to designate coasts, islands, mountains, and the boundaries of political entities. However, some of the products that issue from the scientific decoding of the genome look remarkably like some sorts of geographical maps. For example, low-resolution physical maps made under light microscopy resemble the high resolution photographs made by remote sensing satellites such as SpaceLab. High resolution genomic maps of E coli or phage T4 have an eerie resemblance to the circular mappamundi of the Middle Ages. Yet for the most part, the investigative methods, the physical materials, and the biochemical references of genomic maps are quite unlike geographical maps and mapping. The interminable series of code letters and words that express sequences would never be mistaken for a roadmap. Still, the metaphor is a useful one—it makes concrete and visible a highly complex and elusive structure of matter.

The mapping metaphor is timely. In 1992 an international commemoration recalled the voyage of Christopher Columbus from Spain to the islands of the West Indies. That commemoration aroused interest and controversy about the Age of Exploration during the fifteenth and sixteenth centuries, when adventurers from the nations of Western Europe touched far corners of the globe. Their explorations made new maps possible and made new methods of mapping necessary. The rough charts and descriptions brought home by the explorers stimulated a new science of mapmaking. Ptolemy's long-forgotten theory of mapmaking was rediscovered and scholars such as Mercator and Ortelius devised ways in which the empirical observations of sailors could be translated into abstract but accurate representations. By the middle of the sixteenth century, all the lines on the surface of the globe had been redrawn, new ones added and old ones rendered more accurate.

The maps drawn on paper reflected vast political moves: nations expanded to empires, civilizations became colonies. The economies of some countries were vitalized, of others destroyed. Peoples crossed seas to find freedom and wealth and, in so doing, brought death, disease, and destruction to other peoples. The Age of Exploration, once seen by the historians as an undiluted good for civilization, is now seen either as a disaster or a paradox. Similarly, the age of scientific progress in genetics should be watched with caution: it can bring great good, but it too can cause harm. The remapping of the patient-physician relationship that will accompany advances in genetic science can be for better or worse. Genomic maps will record, not only new scientific knowledge—they will signal social, cultural, and economic revisions in interpersonal relationships and in the institutions of medicine and health care. Some of these revisions will bring great benefit and improvement; others will be problematic and puzzling.

The similarity between the historical events leading to mapping and the modern project of genomic mapping justifies the mapmaking metaphor. But there is a second reason why the metaphor is suitable. Empirical charting and drawing of coasts, mountains, and valleys required a new science, topography. That science used fixed points, situated by surveying instruments or, today, by aerial photography, to calculate with accuracy the dimensions of the mapped surface. Coincidentally, long before topography, ancient philosophers and rhetoricians used the word "topos," meaning "place," to designate the fixed points around which any discourse or argument is arranged. We still require "topics" to guide us through the mixed multitude of facts and assertions that can be brought to any serious discussion of any significant problem. The topics are the fixed points that allow us to put our discourse in some order. If they are well chosen, they reflect the principal features and issues of the problem.

The relationship between physicians and their patients is one such complex area of discourse. That relationship has a long, somewhat obscure history. It is influenced by past traditions and by present institutional structures. It is shaped by conceptions of science and definitions of disease, as well as by conceptions of professionalism and definitions of patienthood. It cannot be described as a simple transaction with quite clearly defined functions and purposes (like, for example, Sartre's famous description of the ticket-taker in the Paris Metro, whose very identity consisted in the punching of tiny cardboards). The relationship, which has certain general and universal features, differs significantly depending on specialties, culture, settings, forms of practice, and economic incentives. Finally, personal styles and personalities render particular relationships quite different from one another.

Discourse about this complex area calls for topics that state the most general and constant features of the relationship. The topics allow not only orderly discussion of the area, but open the way to further analysis and criticism. The purpose of this chapter, then, is to suggest the topics that might delineate the relationship between patients and physicians in an era when genomic information will have become scientifically indispensable and clinically useful. To be more precise, this essay provides more a topology of the relationship than a map: it offers fixed points for description rather than detailed directions for getting around. Still, the metaphor of mapping serves well enough.

Mapping the Medical Relationship

In every map certain very prominent features stand out. If we look at a map of North America, the shape of the continent dominates the map; if we look at a topographical map of Alaska, the mountains of the Alaskan and the Brooks ranges strike our attention. Similarly, the map of the patient-physician relationship has certain characteristics that are both prominent and persisting. These are the essence of the relationship and can be found throughout its history and in every culture. The philosopher and historian of medicine Pedro Lain Entralgo surveys the relationship over diverse times and places and defines it as, "a quasi-dyadic and helpful cooperation, whose purpose is that the patient should achieve the psychosomatic situation we call health."[2] It is dyadic because two persons, one in need of help for physical and/or mental distress and the other offering it, interact in ways that both believe will relieve that distress. It is "quasi-dyadic," because there may be others, ranging from nurses and technicians in our culture to whole villages in other cultures, involved in certain ways in the interaction. This is the essential definition, the most prominent topographical feature, of the relationship.

Around that central feature, many other features cluster. These others are rearranged over time, just as in a geographical map a coastline shifts due to erosion or a new valley is cut by a river or, on a political map, boundaries are redrawn by diplomacy or war. These rearrangements redraw the map of the patient-physician relationship. The map has been redrawn in significant ways several times in the history of Western medicine. A map that would describe the ways in which physicians in fifth-century Greece related to those who sought their help would differ greatly from the map for the medieval French physicians and patients.[3,4] Unfortunately, we do not have enough information to draw these maps in any detail. We can, however, designate some of the fixed points around which richer historical detail could be arranged. In each of those maps, for example, the way in which healing was understood in relation to religion would be a fixed point, allowing historians to accumulate comparative and contrasting information. Similarly, the forms of social and economic life proper to each era would structure the relationship in particular ways. One topic, medical theory, is particularly salient: the ways in which particular eras understood the nature of disease and healing and expressed that in theoretical formulations as well as in practices. Changing theory and practice (the two are not always coordinated or even compatible) would seem to lead almost inevitably to changes in the relationship between healers and the sick. The historical record of the evolution of medical theory is ample, but many gaps remain. It is particularly difficult to trace the relation between theory and practice: to what extent did the theoretical understanding of disease guide the actual decisions and actions of doctors caring for patients? Did modes of healing inspire new theory or theory suggest new modes of healing? It is difficult to answer with any assurance.

However, one such revision of theory is recent enough that we enjoy abundant historical information both about the emergence of theory and the radical modifications of medical practice that ensued. That revision took place during the mid-nineteenth century. Prior to that time, physicians learned about their patient's illness primarily from the patient's own reporting of their symptoms and they linked those reports to ebbs and flows of internal fluids that themselves responded to external, cosmic forces. In almost all ancient medical theory, the patient was a microcosm engulfed in the macrocosm. Interventions were designed to redress imbalances not only within, but between within and without. Often, the physician did not intervene by using the available medical means, such as drugs, bleeding, or cautery, but rather gave advice about how the patient was to change his or her ways. Changes in diet, exercise, place of residence were frequently prescribed to redress the imbalance of humors. There was no direct empirical evidence of internal fluids or humors, at least as they were supposed to function as causes of health and disease. There was no way of proving the causal link between the presumed internal changes and the external influences. There existed no reliable way to link signs and symptoms of illness to the malfunction of discrete organ systems. Astrology was as plausible an explanation of illness as was anatomy.

In the nineteenth century, medical sciences became increasingly capable of relating the patient's signs and symptoms to an organically based pathology. The classical disease of a single microcosmic imbalance fractured into multiple diseases sited in specific organs and caused by specific agents. The patient was no longer a microcosm but rather a site for disease processes. This required a redrawing of the map between patient and physician. In the former era, the physician stood before the patient as a listener, observer, and counselor. In the new age of physiological pathology, the physician gradually became an intervener, seeking out the organic or organismic source of disease and extirpating it. The new physician became able to enter the living body, first by stethoscopic auscultation, then by x-ray and all its radiological and endoscopic successors; the bodily cavities were physically entered by sterile, painless surgery. As the physical boundaries were passed, the relational boundaries changed. Just as the empirical data brought back by the explorers of the Age of Discovery led to a redrawing of the political map of the world, similarly, the new information at the level of theory and of data gathered by nineteenth-century scientific physicians began to force a redrawing of the relational map of physician and patient.

That new map took on the following configuration. It shows a patient presently suffering from an ailment presenting himself or herself to a physician. This differs little or not at all from the traditional way in which the dyadic relation had been initiated (although in the past, persons with access to physicians often approached them for advice about preserving health and avoiding disease and that advice was readily given). However, unlike the past, the physician of the modern era, after listening to the complaint and its history, sets out immediately to verify the physical site of the disease which the signs and symptoms already suggest. Even the techniques of physical diagnosis, which we take so for granted, are the creation of the nineteenth century, in which it became possible to link signs and symptoms in a systematic way to the processes of cellular and organic pathology. The search may start with visual examination and palpation but then is carried on through interventions that probe with instruments and record data that can be interpreted in pathological terms. The thermometer, now a household item, became useful only in the nineteenth century, when calibrations could be related to physical states and the various etiologies of fever were under-stood.[5] The probes of the ancient, medieval, and Renaissance physicians were limited: they felt the pulse, palpated for tumor, rigor, and calor and inspected urine and feces. The modern diagnostic intervention frequently leads to a therapeutic intervention, usually by drugs, surgery, or radiation. The emphasis on intervention in modern medicine, aimed at the precise designation of the etiology of the disease in specific organic lesions, is the most striking feature of the map of modern medicine that began to be drawn in the nineteenth century. The modern descendants of Virchow seek the modern equivalent of cellular pathology; the successors of Koch and Pasteur identify and eradicate noxious microbes and the beneficiaries of the Bayer Company's ability to synthesize drugs from chemicals still prescribe targeted interventions. Physicians still encounter patients in Lain Entralgo's "dyadic cooperation" aimed at the achievement of health. They simply have more expansive understanding and elaborate probes to carry out that cooperation.

Genomic Information

Genomic information will effect many changes in the ways in which we understand the biochemical basis of human development and of health and disease. Put in the most general way, genomic information will increase the specificity with which we can identify and predict the biochemical determinants of developmental and physiological normalcy and abnormality. The inevitable development of disease and the presence of risks for disease, as well as possibilities for prevention, cure, and risk reduction will become much more visible than ever before. New probes, such as fluorescent molecules, once launched in the genomic sea will moor at a specific harbor in the chromosome and from there signal to explorers about the topography of mutations. Those signals will make it possible to link disease and disease risks to the patient's past and project them into the patient's future. These new probes and the science behind them will bring, in my estimation, four major shifts that will move the present boundaries of the patient-physician relationship. The first will shift the relationship from the Present into the Future, the second from Possibility to Actuality, the third from Activity to Contemplation, and the fourth from Duality to Multitude. These are the topics that will define the relationship between the genomic physicians and their patients. These are odd designations on the legend of the new map: I will now attempt to explain why I envision them in the future of genomic medicine.

8

Present to Future

This first shift will be from Present to Future, or more accurately, the drawing of the Future into the Present. In modern medicine, a person becomes a patient at the point when a present ailment manifests itself (I abstract from the broader sense of "patient" that covers the quasi-contractual relationships involved in finding and selecting someone to provide physician services when needed). People come to the doctor with a "presenting complaint." The activities of diagnosis and treatment are usually initiated in this way. Unquestionably, we recognize risks for future disease: chronic hypertension carries risk of cardiac disease and stroke. Unquestionably, we encourage prevention: on discovering hypertension, weight control is advised. Still, the dyadic cooperation usually begins with signs and symptoms responded to by diagnostic and therapeutic interventions. (Hypertension is often found by chance in the course of seeing a doctor for some other problem.)

Genomic information will signal future disease, disease susceptibility, or disease risks. As the molecular basis for single-gene inheritance of common debilitating diseases unfolds, diagnosis and prognosis will collapse into each other. It appears that the first successful voyages of discovery into the genome will lead to the mapping and sequencing of many, and ultimately all, of those conditions known to be monogenic—that is, due to a mutation in a single gene. This will expand the capacity for carrier screening and presymptomatic detection that already exists. This information will give an almost palpable presence in the patient's (or parent's) mind and emotions to many conditions of varying severity that would otherwise not be perceived, felt, or experienced by the affected person for relatively long periods of time. It now is possible for someone to say, "I have Huntington's disease," long before any manifestations of that dread disease will cripple the body. As the genome map becomes more specific, similar statements will be validated for a variety of other serious conditions. The patient's present and future will collapse into each other.

We already know that there are families in which breast cancer, colon cancer, or Alzheimer's disease are inherited in an autosomal dominant fashion. Future disease will become a much more prominent feature of the future patient-physician relationship. Persons could be designated patients in an anticipatory sense. Some with monogenic disorders will be patients without symptoms, but sure to have them in the future. Others, with the genetic patterns associated with polygenic or multifactorial disorders, will be known as a schizophrenic or cardiac or cancer patient long before any illness is felt or any pathology damages the organism; indeed, they may never be affected at all, yet still be marked. Persons will become patients before their time: They will be described in disease terms but "feel fine" and "be fine" for years, perhaps always. Their future, however, will be more vividly present to them and to others than ever before. They will be given a picture of a future self to await, contemplate, and worry about.

Possibility to Actuality

Not only will the Future become Present, but the Possible will become Actual. Modern medicine knows enough about "risk factors" to be able to inform patients with certain characteristics or life styles that they are susceptible to certain diseases and, given the convergence of multiple circumstances, they may sometime become ill. Classic genetics described the patterns of inheritance that constituted risk for disease or for transmission of disease to offspring. Still, the development of actual disease lay in the future and remained a probability, not only in the statistical but in the psychological sense. Genomic information will identify an increasing number of genetic loci in which the presence of a specific DNA sequence, perhaps one of several variant sequences or alleles found at that locus, is associated with susceptibility for a condition, such as cardiovascular disease, cancer, diabetes, or depression. Some of these conditions will be polygenic; others will require environmental and behavioral co-factors; in both cases, the number of these may be vast and their nature obscure.

In the psychology of ordinary life, futures lie in the realm of possibility. Possibility is made up of an infinite number of causal lines, some few of which will converge to make an actuality for individuals. Even when a person clearly knows that they have a lethal disease, such as cancer, the future course of the disease and their eventual death, though certain to happen, remains a possibility, since when and how it happens depends on the haphazard, random convergence of causes, many of which may not in any way be related to their disease. Even more, a prediction of cardiovascular disease due to high cholesterol or lung cancer due to smoking: so much more needs to happen between the presumed stimulus and the eventual response. The threatened person can, and often does, say, "That won't happen to me."

Genomic information will, I estimate, change this ordinary life psychology. Persons will learn, with scientific assurance, that the disease susceptibility is written in the letters of their genome. Certainly, it remains true that the convergence of many factors needed to trigger the disease may not come about and may be avoided by behaviors, but still, the chanciness and luck of the draw that accompany present-day risk assessment will be replaced by the clear mark of the susceptibility in one's very identity. Even though the illness has not yet appeared, it has been found biochemically present: it is an actuality, not a possibility. Even though prediction of clinical manifestations in the individual will not be highly accurate, since it will derive from population data, the reality of risk will be much more tangible. Today these risks are written in abstract numbers that have but remote impact on the way in which persons see themselves; tomorrow these risks will be written in each one's genome, an indelible part of the self. The anticipatory patients will watch themselves and will be watched by physicians for the appearance of disease. Yet physicians may say, "You have x" (as we may say today of a person with the Huntington's mutation, "you have Huntington's disease"), and patients may believe this of themselves. This, of course, may be of benefit, should prevention or early treatment be possible. But, whether beneficial or not, possible disease will become actual, as never before. Just as my genetics are me, so my mutations and the disease that they in some way effect, will be me.

Genomic information should provide not only the diagnostic and prognostic aspects of the patient-physician relationship, but it should also point toward the therapeutic. Many new routes to disease prevention will be opened up. Routes toward the therapy of disease will also be plotted. Indeed, experiments in gene replacement therapy have already been initiated. We can glimpse ways in which genomic information can guide and enhance current pharmacotherapy. Still, the theoretical potential for therapy is not likely to be realized soon in any broad, much less universal way. Unquestionably, this has always been true of medicine: many diseases have been recognized and even well understood without the faintest hope of curing or changing their course. This became dramatically true in the mid-nineteenth century, when medical science tore the veil of ignorance between disease and organic pathology. So much became known about the causes of disease and so little was available to treat it effectively that "therapeutic nihilism" became the prevailing medical philosophy. Gradually, with the appearance of effective pharmaceuticals and efficient surgery, this nihilism was converted into a therapeutic activism, which continues to be the dominant approach to disease. Even though many disorders defy effective medical intervention, intervention of some sort has become mandatory. Indeed, it has become a common clinical joke that the wise sen-

---

11

ior physician must frequently admonish the junior doctors, "don't do something, just stand there!"

Genomic information will exaggerate the gap between diagnosis and therapy. Today, in the practice of clinical genetics, the major product of the patient-physician or counselor encounter is information. Persons who have had a child affected by a known genetic disease seek advice about the risk of having another such child in the future. A few persons who know that a genetic disease exists in their family pedigree, or who are members of an ethnic group at particular risk of a disease, come for assurance that they are not inheritors. But, unlike most of modern medicine, the interventions, other than the diagnostic ones such as amniocentesis, are few, and the direct therapies almost non-existent. The information provided is used primarily for procreative planning.

As genomic information about disease susceptibility becomes more common, clinical genetics will acquire a new sort of information. It will deal, not only with procreative predictions, but with predictions about the life and life style of the patient who seeks the information. What the internist now diagnoses at the presentation of symptoms, the medical geneticist may be able to diagnose on the examination of cells obtained within a few days after conception, or at any time during pregnancy and early life. It is not bizarre to imagine a time when a future health "history" might be worked out from an embryonic biopsy. Medical geneticists will have the ability to become premonitory cardiologists or oncologists. Since they will have no therapy to apply, since no disease has yet appeared, and may never, they will have to devise new forms of doctoring. They will become watchful waiters, and evaluators of the many health events that might herald the onset of the predicted disease, constant advisors about life styles and choices that might reduce the threat.

Scientia Activa to *Scientia Contemplativa*

This suggests a third shift of boundaries on the map of the patient-physician relationship: a shift from what medieval philosophers described as a *Scientia Activa* to a *Scientia Contemplativa*; from an active, practical science to a theoretical, speculative one. Modern medicine is predominantly a *Scientia Activa*, a collection of diagnostic and therapeutic actions that start in the logic of clinical judgment and terminate in interventions. Modern medicine reluctantly acknowledges the presence of untreatable disease, but assumes that at some future time the untreatable will be successfully treated. Genomic information, however, will announce the presence or the possibility of disease without the application of the logic of clinical judgment and for which therapeutic intervention may be unavailable. Lain Entralgo's statement of the traditional goal of the patient-physician relationship, "to achieve the psychosomatic state we call health," may very often be beyond the powers of the physician of the genomic era. We have already seen this in one of modern genetics' first clinical triumphs, siting the locus of Huntington's disease. We now know the genesis of a devastating disease about which we can do absolutely nothing. Indeed, at the very beginning of the science of molecular genetics forty years ago, the genetics of sickle-cell disease were unraveled and no cure has yet appeared. Finally, many genetic diagnoses will be made in the fetus in utero which, as a consequence, will be aborted and thus cut off from the "psychosomatic state we call health."

As the mapped genome opens up broad vistas of information, it will, in a strange sense, return to medicine's impotent past. Genomic information, then, will promise many means of cure and prevention, but those means will remain ideas in the minds of inquiring scientists for years before some of them are transformed into therapeutic tools in the hands of the physician. We will learn much about the interactions between genes, between gene products and between genetic structures and environmental factors. Prognosis, the ancient art of predicting the natural course of disease, is likely to be the principal clinical beneficiary of genomic information, at least for the foreseeable future. Today's medicine, a *Scientia Activa*, may become tomorrow a *Scientia Contemplativa*: many diseases will be understood more radically at the molecular level than ever before, but the disease course cannot be changed, at least with current knowledge; thus it can only be expected, watched and wondered about, by both patient and physician.

The new map, then, contains one dimension, the shift from active to contemplative, that revives an approach to medicine that modern medical activists had thought long past. It also contains three dimensions that were not prominent features of the old: a concentration on the future, an emphasis on potentiality, and the final topic I wish to discuss, the expansion from duality to multitude. Just as the "cooperation" that linked the dyad will be more a watchful waiting than an active intervention and the "psychosomatic condition called health" will be defined as future rather than present, as potential rather than actual disease, so the "quasi-dyad" of physician and patient will become a veritable multiplicity of persons, all involved in the interaction.

13

Duality to Multitude

The fourth major shift in the patient-physician relationship will be from Duality to Multitude. Modern medicine is, as Lain Entralgo expressed, a duality between a patient and a physician. He even characterized it as a species of *philia*—that is, friendship. Genomic information will push back the bounds of that duality into wider communities or populations. Genetic information by definition ties an individual into his or her heritage and to his or her heirs. The diseases linked to genetic loci flow through families from generation to generation. The individual who stands before his or her physician seeking information and help is, in the genetic view, an instance of a group linked together through social institutions such as marriage and heritage and through shared biochemical characteristics. This is vividly illustrated by the practice of clinical geneticists whose first diagnostic act is not auscultation and palpation but the drawing of a family pedigree. It is manifested in one of the first scientific techniques based on recombinant DNA technology devised to search out genetic defects, the RFLP linkage maps: whole families and different generations must be drawn into the diagnostic process. We even see this in the termination of pregnancy following prenatal diagnosis: a potential heir is eliminated. Decisions to procreate will be informed by more extensive medical information derived not only from the parent, but from the kinship. Information about disease will pertain, not only to the presenting patient, but to others to whom that patient is linked by kinship. Do they have the right to that information? How will it affect their lives, their reproductive choices, their views of themselves and their parents? Are they as much patients as the person whom the physician now sees? Physicians of the future will have to see beyond the presenting patient to the cohort around the patient, working with the complex relationships, experiences, and emotions of the many who are linked together at the molecular level.

We also can glimpse the presence of others, genetically unrelated, but intensely interested in the individual or family under investigation: insurers, employers, public health officials, police, government. Individual risk profiles will find their way into many computers and file drawers: the intrinsic difficulty of interpreting them accurately will be ignored as they become useful instruments for sorting out the healthy from the ill, the good risks from the bad, the safe from the dangerous, the cost-effective from the costly. More and more, a large population will stand around each patient, providing essential information, posing possibilities for prevention, and seeking out previously private information for purposes of social or economic utility. The many problems about confidentiality and privacy of information that have been noted in genomic ethics are based upon the reality of a genome shared among a kinship, but also upon the usefulness that the information has to many persons beyond that kinship. The duality of the modern relation between physician and patient will widen into a broad community. The Duality will become a Multitude.

This new map will reveal the presence of another population, just as the maps of explorers noted the places in which indigenous people dwelt. The new population will be the vast number of "unpatients" that genomic information will identify. An "unpatient" is a person who does not now suffer from a disease condition that debilitates them or is even felt by them. They are not in need of, nor can they be given, any treatment. Thus, they are not, in any proper sense of the word, "patients." At the same time, they have entered the medical world through screening or some other genetic diagnostic process. They have been identified as having the relevant gene for a monogenic condition or the genetic background for susceptibility or risk for a polygenic and multifactorial condition. They have a disease in potentiality which may or may not manifest itself to greater or lesser degree. And they know this (or their parents know this) with assurance, if not with certainty. Thus, being designated as part of the world of medicine and being an object of medical interest, they are patients. Persons in this situation might be called "unpatients." They are somewhat like the vampires in old horror movies who were neither alive nor dead and were called "the undead." Many of the features of medicine and health care will pertain to them; many others, particularly the ability to offer Lain Entralgo's "helping cooperation," will not be available. Yet, they, fated with this knowledge about their future, will want and need to be watched.

This has implications for access to health care. The new population of genetically diagnosable unpatients is of unknown proportions. At present, the numbers seeking genetic diagnosis are relatively small: for the most part, they are persons with known high risks of rare conditions. The numbers of trained medical geneticists and genetic counselors are small. But with each advance in diagnostic capability the population will grow and the need for providers will increase. We already have the instrument that may propel the first wave of that onslaught: the diagnostic ability to detect cystic fibrosis by carrier screening and prenatal testing. This autosomal recessive disease affects one out of every 2,500 babies born in the United States; more than 8 million Americans may be carriers of the gene. The population at risk of being carriers of cystic fibrosis are all persons of Caucasian descent. Thus, the prospect of an effective program to detect the carriers of the gene and the victims of this lethal disease raises daunting problems of scope, design, and cost.[6]

Beyond carrier and diagnostic testing for specific genetic diseases, devising genetic tests for susceptibility to more common diseases will become a major scientific and commercial endeavor. Even though any test of this sort, scientifically sophisticated though it may be, will be difficult to interpret, people are likely to think it a good thing. For example, a gene on chromosome 17 carries a mutation that predisposes some women to breast and ovarian cancer. One in 200–400 American women may be carriers of that mutation. The authors of a paper discussing this matter comment, "The prevalence of BRCA1 mutation female carriers, themselves at approximately 85% risk of developing breast/or ovarian cancer, far exceeds that of any genetic disorder for which presymptomatic screening is currently available. This issue alone raises significant social and economic concerns about the feasibility of population-based screening ... (which) is likely to be the first widespread presymptomatic genetic test that finds its way into general medical practice."[7] Given the current concern about these diseases, the desire for such a test is likely to be high among women. If limited to women over age 18 who have a clear history of breast cancer in their families, some 600,000 women might benefit from the test. However, even when family history is unknown or uncertain, many more women and their doctors might desire, and order, the test. Thus, the demand for the test could be vast, although it might often be inappropriate. The genetic test itself must be attended by counseling, should lead to regular surveillance for disease, and may lead to prophylactic surgery. Much more research will be required—and demanded by women—to understand the path from genetic mutation to actual disease and to devise preventive measures short of prophylactic mastectomy. This implies a massive expansion of services and costs, just as it opens opportunities for commercial and medical exploitation of this vast market.

Genomic information, then, will gradually bring diagnostic capabilities that allow for widespread screening of large populations for numerous conditions. The screening procedures will have to be defined with care. Programs will have to be mounted efficiently and effectively, and screening will have to be accompanied by counseling and by followup. Those persons discovered to be positive for the condition being screened for will need treatment, if treatment is available, or will have to be counseled, followed, watched, and treated for the disease when it manifests itself. Almost all of this activity will be added on to our present health care system. Indeed, some cases of possible disease will be prevented by knowledge which allows heterozygotes to decide whether to avoid procreation; others will be prevented by decisions to abort based upon prenatal diagnosis. Even then, in both cases, effective testing and counseling will add new responsibilities to our current health services, and abortion services will have to be more freely and widely available than they are at present. Quite different forms of service, encompassing families, communities, and populations, will have to be invented. Many of the duties in these different forms of service, such as management of familial testing, are not within the current repertoire of most physicians and may have to be added or assigned to new sorts of professionals. In general, the new population of unpatients, from the diagnosed fetus to the adult anticipating the onset of disease, will become real, if partial, participants in the world of health care and call for new and expanded services.

Naturally, the advent of new, expanded services raises questions of access, utilization, and cost. It is presently unclear how such services would be mounted, organized, and paid for. It is possible that many persons might have access to certain levels of genetic services, such as a population screening program, and not to other levels of service, such as counseling or treatment. This already has happened in the effort to screen for sickle cell disease in a population that was in general medically underserved. Individuals positive for the trait or the disease were identified but, once identified, were often left as remote from education, counseling, and care as they had been before. The new powers of molecular medicine challenge the structure of the health care system as it presently exists.

The New Map Evaluated

This, then, is my new map of the patient-physician relationship that will be drawn as the exploration of the human genome proceeds. The current map of a duality dealing actively with a present disorder will be redrawn to show a community contemplating a future disorder or probability thereof. Obviously, the old and the new maps overlap at many points: there are within the current repertoire of medicine situations which look much like the situations of the future. Obviously, as well, future situations will often be quite similar to the present. Yet, I am suggesting that a major shift will take place. The maps of the sixteenth century did sharpen many of the geographical boundaries; yet these were but minor shifts. Much more importantly, they revealed "theres" that had been previously unknown and showed how it was possible to get from here to there in previously unsuspected ways. These were the major shifts.

The mapping of the human genome, then, will require a remapping of the relationship between physician and patient. Unlike the mapping of the genome, which is a scientific voyage of discovery, the remapping of the relationship is a political adventure. It will require diplomacy and may result in revolutions in social institutions, legal provisions, and economic arrangements. New claims of rights and duties will emerge. Above all, just as when political boundaries are redrawn, loyalties and allegiances will be challenged. The bond that has tightly linked physician and patient for many centuries will be stretched within the emerging network of the multitudes to whom genomic information is valuable. The traditional ethical features of the relationship, such as the definition of the fiduciary relationship and the duties of confidentiality, may have to be redesigned in some respects and strengthened in others.

The new map of the patient-physician relationship will reveal that the structures of health care services and financing that were built on the old map are outmoded for the new world. New scientific information will be translated into new procedures, at the levels of populations and of individuals. New patients will be discovered and the "unpatients" will come into view. New services will be designed, requiring many professionals to staff them. The services will cost money, which must be paid from some pocket, public or private. Some savings may be realized by the prevention or early treatment of disease, but those savings may be offset by the costs of population screening and by increases in volume caused by the "unpatients." And, inevitably, in a health care system like the American one, profits will be made that will increase costs and contribute little to the quality and efficiency of the system. Thus, the new map of the patient-physician relationship will soon be filled with newly designed systems, or at least, the need and demand for them, just as the empty spaces of the discoverers' maps rapidly filled with towns and cities.

The shifts described here are, like all major changes in social and institutional life, a mixture of positive and negative. Genomic information promises significant therapeutic possibilities, but we must not delude ourselves by believing that they will come quickly or that they will be universal. Similarly, the shifts from the highly interventional *Scientia Activa* to something more like a *Scientia Contemplativa* may not be all bad, given the notable power of intervention to harm or to do nothing for the patient. Finally, the shift from duality to multitude might press modern medicine out of the excessive individualism that ignores social and community responsibilities. Each shift, like each discovery of new lands and each movement of peoples from an old world into a new, will bring a mix of benefits and burdens, goods and evils.

It has been said that modern physicians treat the pathology rather than the patient. This accusation arises from the unquestionably beneficial discoveries of the nineteenth century that allowed physicians to find pathology in cells and organs and to trace its causes to invading microbes. The genomic physician will go even deeper, stalking disease down to the molecular—to mutations in nucleotide sequences. This may exaggerate the unfortunate tendency to reductionism, whereby the physician fails to recognize that a diseased heart or liver resides in a human person. The genomic physician may become so enthralled by the code within the chromosome that the patient moves even further out of sight.

However, the genomic physician may be saved from that error precisely by the other shifts in the relationship. The diagnosis that reveals a future disease or its possibility, and involves necessarily a community around the patient, may force physicians to look up from the physical site of the disease to the full context in which it will appear. They will have to consider, with the patient, the future and the potential. They will have to watch and wait, with the patient. They will have to counsel about the implications of choices. They will have to link the patient with the kinship and protect the patient from others who would use genetic information to the patient's detriment. The genomic physician may be forced to live in a world larger than the organ system and the chromosome.

It may be that genomic medicine has the potential to be more human and humane than contemporary medicine, since the changes in the patient-physician relationship that I have envisioned reflect profound features of what theologians like to call "the humanum," the radical features of human nature and the human condition. Human beings, more than any other animal we know, live from the past into the future, contemplate those futures and dwell in the midst of multitudes. To the extent that patients and physicians become more conscious of these features of their relationship, to that extent should the relationship be humanized. This is something to hope for.

The ships that sailed from Europe five centuries ago not only mapped the world; they inaugurated social, political, and economic events that radically changed humankind's view of itself and nations' views of their destinies. The map of the New World was not drawn only by Columbus,

Drake, and Magellan. It was also drawn by the rulers, Philip II and Elizabeth I, sending brave colonists and savage exploiters who together created a new political map. It was drawn as well by theologians, such as Francisco Vitoria and Bartolomeo de las Casas, who expounded, in academic and polemic terms, on the new ethical imperatives and responsibilities of rulers, settlers, and explorers. The rapidly redrawn map of discovery and colonization depicted areas of glorious achievement and other areas of deplorable tragedy. The discoveries that will lead to the mapping of the genome will have similar dramatic effects on our perception of our nature and our relationships with each other. We will inevitably rejoice in some of these effects and regret others.

We must proceed with these explorations but, as one clinical geneticist, Neil Holzmann, has said, we must proceed with caution.[8] A dictum of St. Thomas Aquinas serves as an annotation to Dr. Holzman's warning. Centuries ago, the theologian said about caution, by which he meant not timidity but carefulness, "caution is required because human behavior is so complex that good and evil are inextricably mixed: the prudent man cannot avoid evil altogether, but he should be careful to avoid by foresight the common pitfalls so that as little harm as possible is done."[9] As the secrets of the genome are unraveled, human good and evil will appear: let us avoid by foresight the common pitfalls so that more good than harm comes of this extraordinary effort to expand the boundaries of human knowledge.

Notes

Support for the writing of this article was provided in part by a grant from the National Center for Human Genome Research, National Institutes of Health, HG004777.

1. Watson, J., Zinder N., *New York Times*, Oct. 13, 1990, p. 14.

2. Lain Entralgo, P., *Doctor and Patient*, trans. Frances Partridge, New York: McGraw-Hill, 1968, p. 152.

3. Edelstein, L., "The Hippocratic physician," in *Ancient Medicine*, Baltimore: Johns Hopkins University Press, 1967.

4. Siraisi, N., *Medieval and Early Renaissance Medicine*, Chicago: University of Chicago Press, 1990.

5. Reiser, S., *Medicine and the Reign of Technology*, New York: Cambridge University Press, 1978.

6. Wilfond B. S., Fost, N., "The cystic fibrosis gene: Medical and social implications for heterozygote detection," *JAMA*, 1990; 263: 2777-83.

20

7. Biesecker B. B., Boehnke M., Calzone K., et al., "Genetic counseling for families with inherited susceptibility to breast and ovarian cancer," *JAMA*, 1993; 269: 1970–74.

8. Holzman, N., *Proceed with Caution*, Baltimore: Johns Hopkins University Press, 1989.

9. Aquinas, Thomas, *Summa Theologiae* II-II, 47, 16, New York and London: McGraw-Hill, 1965.

Two

Educating Clinicians
about Genetics

Vincent M. Riccardi

A treatise on Beethoven's symphonies is *about* his music; it is not a performance of that music. This chapter is about the education of clinicians; it is not an effort to provide that education. Nonetheless, the material has been written for clinicians as well as educators and policy makers. For the *clinicians*, I wish to convince them both that medical genetics is a routine part of primary and secondary care and that new developments in molecular genetics make genetics more rather than less accessible to them and their patients. For the *educators*, I wish to encourage them to share the wealth of old and new genetic facts and principles, respecting the significance of the Human Genome Project (HGP) and changes in what it means to be a clinician. For the *policy makers*, I wish to impress them that the strategies are meaningful, clear and straighforward.

A recent editorial entitled, "Science education: Who needs it?" (Hackerman 1992), has already introduced some of the important issues. I cite it because its emphasis on *"public literacy* with respect to science and technology" (emphasis added) leads to an equally strong case being made for *professional literacy* in the sciences and technologies that impinge directly on the day-to-day activities of clinicians. Genetics is a paradigm of such a science and the HGP is a superb vehicle for affording *genetic literacy* to the general public and to professionals, especially clinicians.

What most of us have in mind when we refer to a *clinician* is a physician who essentially devotes his or her career to direct interaction with patients. A broader definition would also allow for practitioners who perform similar activities on a part-time basis and for those who do so other than as physicians; for example, registered nurses, nurse practitioners, dentists, chiropractors, and so on. Although ultimately all such clinicians need to understand the nature and consequences of the HGP, in this chapter I will focus on clinicians in the first, more restricted sense.

A key aspect of the HGP is that genetics is changing, and, in turn, so is the way genetics can be used by clinicians. But clinicians are also changing. For example, the clinician is increasingly called upon to demonstrate more financial and business acumen. I see major changes in the roles clinicians play, especially their emergence as literal *managers* of health care planning and delivery, making more decisions on behalf of patients without the benefit of hands-on contact.

Cost-consciousness will be a key aspect of the clinician-manager's role. Thus, as clinicians employ the benefits of progress in human genetics, they must simultaneously acknowledge the financial expense of doing so; they must show a significant financial value as well as a clinical benefit. Bringing the new genetics to clinicians must also acknowledge that they are new clinicians. To be effective, the two sources of novelty should complement each other.

There's an old saw that "physicians do the right thing and managers do things right." There is a certain amount of utility in that aphorism: clinicians have always been expected to do "the right thing" in discharging their duties to patients, regardless of the obstacles, financial or otherwise. The obstacles were, by and large, superimposed externalities that the clinicians, the patients, and their families conspired to minimize or obviate. Managers, on the other hand, either imposed the obstacles or were directed by the clinicians to assist in surmounting them.

Scope of the Task

What is genetics? Up through the 1970s, genetic disorders were considered rare curiosities, the major responsibility for which fell to self-styled medical geneticists. During the 1980s, the notion of rare curiosities continued, but the medical geneticists themselves had increased in number and were assisted by new classes of health professionals, including Ph.D. medical geneticists, nurse geneticists, and genetic associates, later to be called genetic counselors. In parallel with this increased visibility and sophistication among clinicians, research became increasingly focused on identifying and analyzing the genes themselves. In addition, by 1990, prenatal diagnosis had become an integral part of routine medical care, with severe legal and financial penalties for failure to use it under certain circumstances.

Genetic principles as they applied in traditional genetic counseling also became relevant to the origin, progression, and treatment of cancer, and even to the diagnosis of nongenetic diseases, particularly infections of various types, not the least of which has been AIDS. For example, there is now the ability to diagnose bladder cancer from DNA analysis of cells contained in urine (Sidransky et al., 1991) and the ability to diagnose colon cancer in stool specimens (Sidransky et al., 1992). In short, genetics has been transformed from esoterica to the mundane: every branch of medicine, every level of clinician has some need to be familiar with genetic principles and their application. In addition, policy makers, those who manage clinicians, and clinicians who manage the business of their private or collective practices, need to take into account consequences of the new genetics, both for its impact on patients and their families and for the costs and savings it engenders.

How much do clinicians need to know? How can we best make that knowledge accessible and meaningful? The HGP provides a unique opportunity for answering these and related questions.

Goals of Clinician Genetic Education

The goals of an education program aimed at clinicians should have three elements: an increase in *background knowledge*, an increase in the ability to make sound *business management decisions*, and an increase in the ability to make sound *clinical decisions*.

Background Knowledge

Even if we did not expect clinicians to make frequent or critical decisions based on genetic principles or genetic data, continuing medical education programs, journal articles and book chapters, colleagues and patients themselves increasingly require clinicians to be familiar with modern genetic precepts. Genetics is an important and growing part of the present medical milieu. One might even say that being a competent, modern clinician is impossible without substantial familiarity with genetics.

24

Business Management Decisions

On one side of the coin, the application of clinical genetic principles is based on specificity to the finest degree. In one type of setting, a clinical diagnosis is already known, but more precision is needed. It is not enough to know that a child has cystic fibrosis: for prenatal diagnosis in subsequent pregnancies of the child's parents and, perhaps, for estimating prognosis, identification and characterization of the paired mutant genes are necessary. It is not enough to know that the patient has chronic myelogenous leukemia: to determine prognosis and treatment, we must know the details of the underlying genetic changes (somatic mutations). Alternatively, in another type of setting, genetic precision can be used to screen for particular disorders; for example, the prenatal diagnosis of trisomy 21, keying off maternal age. In screening scenarios, however, only a small percentage of individuals tested will have a positive result; much more often than not, the test will yield negative results.

On the other side of the coin is recognition that the relevant tests are generally labor-intensive and utilize sophisticated technical equipment: they are expensive. Given increasing pressures to minimize expenses, when does it become realistic to use this technology? And who makes such decisions? Increasingly, "bedside" clinicians have been replaced as decision-makers by managers in the health care system who weigh the costs and benefits.

Clinical Decisions

There are two kinds of clinical decision-making: those decisions implemented *directly* for the patient (e.g., prescription of a medication, ordering a laboratory test); and those that are made on behalf of the patient, essentially *channeling* the patient to another clinician (e.g., obtaining a genetics consultation). By and large, the vast majority of clinicians have chosen the latter approach, passing decision-making on to the geneticist. I believe this will change as the increased knowledge from the HGP and other medical genetic research requires all clinicians to make genetic decisions directly for their patients. The range and frequency of such decisions will become so great that displacement to a clinical geneticist for each instance of decision-making will be impossible.

Recognizing the distinction between direct implementation and channeling for genetic disorders should encourage clinicians to take a more active role in their patients' genetic health care, and not hand them over to a geneticist. The latter will simply be overwhelmed: not because of an increase in the total number of genetic diseases, but an increase in the recognition of genetic diseases for which meaningful intervention is possible.

Direct Implementation

If the clinician is already aware of, or newly identifies, a genetic condition (or the risk for it), he or she might then clarify directly the heritability (i.e., recurrence) risks, order appropriate diagnostic tests, or both. As we learn more about genetic diseases, patients for whom such a direct disposition is required will become increasingly common.

Channeling

In other instances, the diagnosis will be so arcane, unclear, or complex that immediately channeling the patient to a geneticist or another specialist might be more prudent. For example, a disorder characterized by diffuse muscular weakness might first require input from a neurologist, whether or not a geneticist is ultimately consulted.

Imperatives for Clinician Genetic Education

Traditional Clinical Imperatives

The traditional medical imperative for a person with or at risk for a genetic disorder has been to minimize the person's suffering in relatively general and nonspecific ways (e.g., institutionalize patients with mental retardation, or merely estimate the time until death for a patient with cancer). As genetic disorders have been more precisely delineated during the twentieth century (e.g., Down syndrome, phenylketonuria), the very surfeit of diagnoses has led, through the traditional approach, to the emphasis on channeling the patient to those professionals most likely to sort through the maze of often overlapping disorders and widely different genetic mechanisms. We are now at that stage wherein it *appears* that the clinician's main, if not sole, responsibility is merely to know when to refer to a clinical geneticist. This approach is changing. Clinicians will soon have the tools to make the appropriate diagnoses on their own.

Technological Imperatives

The basis for such an assertion is current technological research exemplified by the HGP: knowledge of the human genome will soon provide a basis for identifying both the "normal" (or, in the geneticist's jargon, the "wild type") genes at any given locus, as well as the most common mutant alleles. *Much as infectious disease is now readily classified into different types* (i.e., those due to fungi, bacteria, mycoplasmas, prions, viruses, etc.), *on the basis of which the clinician can make sophisticated decisions directly for the patient, soon he or she will be able to do so for the patient with or at risk for a genetic disorder.*

Technology has also allowed us to extend what we mean by genetic disease. The genetic basis of cancer is now standard knowledge, whether the genetic factors or changes are inherited or occur subsequently (e.g., as somatic mutations or viral insertion). This knowledge of the genetic underpinnings of cancer is increasingly the basis for precise diagnosis, prognosis, and prescribing treatment. Moreover, genetic technology will become the standard for screening large populations, exemplified by the ability to identify specific mutations in cancer cells in urine sediment and in colon cancer cells in stool specimens. Clinicians need to understand the basis for such tests, when to use them, and how to interpret the results.

The Human Genome Project Imperatives

The HGP embodies a claim that genetics will be the key to practicing medicine in the twenty-first century. Whether the genetic changes are inborn or acquired (i.e., as somatic mutations or viral insertions), whether they are expressed morphologically, immunologically, or biochemically, being aware of these changes and understanding how they influence health is the key to the future, for which we must prepare now.

On the one hand, our older, classical understanding of genetics is being made more useful now that genes (loci, alleles, mutations) are not mere abstractions. The HGP is transforming them into palpable elements of normal and abnormal physiology. On the other hand, genetic research shows us that classical genetic approaches do not account for all the genetic perturbations that underlie human suffering. The HGP is helping us make these otherwise arcane phenomena more readily understood. For example, the expression of a gene may be different, depending on whether it is inherited from the mother or father (genomic imprinting), and sometimes both copies of a given chromosome derive from one parent and not from both parents, as expected from classical genetics (uniparental disomy).

The Relevance of
Clinician Genetic Education

Old and New Mechanisms of Disease

Normal gene function is compromised when the gene's structure is perturbed (i.e., so that it cannot be transcribed, the amount of transcription is abnormal, or the final gene product is dysfunctional) or the gene is literally lost (i.e., deleted). Disturbances of gene structure can result from physical rearrangements of the DNA, some of which are apparent by doing chromosome analysis and some of which require molecular methodologies for demonstration. Or some gene disturbances may be inferred from yet poorly understood processes during gamete formation or embryologic development (e.g., genomic imprinting). Classical genetics has focused on the former, fixed changes (i.e., mutations) in genes, and, as well, changes that are heritable or germinal.

Modern genetics now gives increasing importance to somatic mutations, the role of externally introduced (i.e., viral) DNA, functional changes in genes, and abnormal chromosome segregation. My intention here is not to outline all elements of the "new genetics," but rather to show that classical genetics fails to account for all genetic mechanisms at play in the causation of human disease. The point is, genetic research has made things simpler and more immediate for the clinician and, as well, more complex. Clinicians will progress to accept more responsibility for the former and rely on medical geneticists only for the latter.

Genomic Imprinting

Genomic imprinting (Hall, 1991; Engel et al., 1991; Hall, 1992) is the phenomenon whereby the expression of a gene (normal or mutant) is influenced by the sex of the parent from whom it was inherited. For example, it appears that the expression of genes on the proximal long arm of chromosome 15 may result in the Prader-Willi syndrome if they are derived from the mother, but in the Angelman syndrome if they are derived from the father. How this effect is mediated is unknown, but perhaps the number of methyl groups incorporated into the DNA of the involved genes may be the explanation. Genomic imprinting may also account for a disorder's variation from one generation to another, some features being more prominent if the mutation is passed through the mother and other features being more prominent if passed through the father. The propensity for a gene to contribute to the development of some cancers may also be influenced by genomic imprinting; for example, Wilms tumor (Ferguson-Smith et al., 1991) or paraganglioma (Heutink et al., 1992). This consideration is obviously important in counseling families.

Uniparental Disomy

Uniparental disomy refers to an individual inheriting both copies (homologues) of a given chromosome from the same parent, instead of one chromosome from each parent (Engel et al., 1991). There are two types of uniparental disomy, depending on whether the two homologues so inherited represent both members of the donating parent's chromosome pair or a double presence of one member of the pair. For example, if a child inherits both copies of chromosome 7 from the mother, the latter may have contributed both of her chromosomes 7 (heterodisomy) or two copies of one of them (isodisomy). In one of the first reported cases of uniparental disomy (Spence et al., 1988), the child had cystic fibrosis on the basis of inheriting the two copies of his mother's chromosome 7 bearing the cystic fibrosis mutation (uniparental isodisomy); the father of the child was not a carrier for cystic fibrosis.

Amplification and Monoallelic Expression

Amplification and monoallelic expression (Zhang & Tycko, 1992) also depart from the expectations based on classical genetics. Increases in the size of a gene (amplification), thereby altering the nature or amount of its expression, is known in several settings. In certain cancers, amplification of one or more genes has been appreciated for years, most notably for segments of the short arm of chromosome 1 in neuroblastomas. More recently, amplifications of repeating units of the fragile-X syndrome gene have been demonstrated, with the revelation that this increase in size explains, at least in part, how the gene manifests itself in clinical terms (Rousseau et al., 1991; Caskey et al., 1992; Harper et al., 1992). A similar finding has also been identified for Steinert myotonic dystrophy (Caskey et al., 1992; Mahadevan et al., 1992). And, finally, literal duplication of a single gene can lead to a specific Mendelian disease, as has been demonstrated for Charcot-Marie-Tooth disease type 1A, the locus for which is on the short arm of chromosome 17 (Lupski et al., 1992). That is, a change in the gene's make-up is not necessary, as disease may result from merely an increase in the number of genes from two to three.

Diagnostic Approaches

The diagnosis and treatment of infectious diseases cannot be left to the specialist in such disorders. The development of vaccines for polio and other common infectious disorders may have derived from the work of infectious disease specialists, but the implementation of strategies to eradicate polio occurs at the primary care level. *Likewise for genetic disorders: their diagnosis and treatment cannot be left to geneticists.* Here the emphasis is on diagnosis. Historically, the diagnosis of genetic diseases has often been deferred to clinical geneticists capitalizing on a specialized clinical acumen. But this approach reflects a reliance on clinical criteria for diagnosis.

For some relatively small number of genetic disorders, appreciation of the disorder's pathogenesis allowed for appreciation of abnormal metabolites (e.g., phenylketonuria) or elucidation of an aberrant gene product (e.g., sickle cell hemoglobinopathy); the presence of either could be used as an alternative criterion for diagnosis. The ability to identify aberrant genes (mutations) themselves has dramatically altered the prospects for accurate diagnosis. For example, although we do not yet understand how the NF-1 gene product, neurofibromin, leads to that disorder's lesions, mutations in the NF-1 gene can be used to confirm the clinical diagnosis of that disorder. Similarly, changes in the number or nature of cancer-associated genes (oncogenes and tumor suppressor genes) serve to diagnose a wide spectrum of malignancies.

Several techniques or approaches are especially noteworthy and the practicing clinician will need to become familiar with them. The first is the ability to characterize either the mutant gene itself, or, if this is not feasible, to track the mutant gene in a family through *genetic linkage*, using patterns of DNA profiles as a marker for the disorder. DNA from an individual is purified and treated with an enzyme that cuts it into various lengths. The lengths of the fragments are determined by the number of sites in the DNA sensitive to the enzyme (cut-sites) and the number of DNA base-pairs between the cut-sites. The fragments are then separated from each other in a sieve-like gel and the fragments for a specific gene (locus) are identified by using DNA that has been radioactively labeled. The labeled DNA, or marker, attaches to the sieved DNA that is similar (complementary) to it. The pattern of fragment sizes so identified represents the individual's DNA for one or two alleles at the locus being studied. This *Southern blot restriction fragment length polymorphism approach* (Risch & Devlin, 1992) has been very fruitful, for example, for three very common disorders, sickle cell anemia, cystic fibrosis and NF-1.

A second approach starts with a sample of one or only a very few cells and increases the amount of selected DNA sequences that may then be analyzed utilizing ordinary techniques; for example, Southern blot analysis. This amplification technique, *polymerase chain reaction* (PCR), is the basis for "DNA fingerprinting" for forensic purposes (Risch & Devlin, 1992), for rapid molecular prenatal diagnosis (e.g., cystic fibrosis), and for the cancer screening procedures alluded to above.

Also related to cancer investigations is a third technique, analysis of "*loss of heterozygosity*" (LOH) in tumor specimens (Devilee et al., 1991). We know that certain genes (loci) are consistently involved in the origin and progression of various cancers (e.g., the Harvey ras oncogene in bladder cancer, the p53 tumor suppressor gene in colon cancer). If, for one of these loci, an individual has two distinct alleles defined by either of the approaches just described (and occasionally others as well), it is possible to demonstrate a loss of one of these alleles in the cancer tissue. While this loss does not explain the whole story (e.g., the remaining allele is likely to be a mutant form), the LOH approach has made it possible to identify readily a wide array of oncogenes and tumor suppressor genes contributing to both common and rare forms of cancer and facilitate their diagnosis. It might also be possible to treat some disease by replacing a deficient or mutated tumor suppressor gene (Marshall, 1991).

A fourth technique, *in situ hybridization*, utilizes labeled complementary DNA, as with the Southern blot approach, but this time the marker is used to identify where it attaches along the length of intact chromosomes, as opposed to fragments of DNA. The label, moreover, can be radioactive or a fluorescent dye. When fluorescent-dye-labeled markers are used to study chromosomes, we speak of fluorescent in situ hybridization, or "FISH." This approach is very useful for identifying the loss or gain of whole chromosomes (Hultan et al., 1991) or chromosomal portions involved in various types of structural abnormalities (e.g., translocation, deletion, inversion). One type of FISH uses markers that identify repeating sequences of base pairs, each sequence specific for a given chromosome, such that the whole chromosome appears to be "painted" by the marker. By using different-colored fluorochromes for different chromosomes, exchanges between two or more chromosomes can be readily identified, including exchanges not identifiable by ordinary cytogenetics methods.

One special diagnostic approach that is unlikely to be feasible without data on large portions of the human genome is "*fetal cell rescue*." Fetal cell rescue involves isolating fetal cells from the maternal circulation during early pregnancy and testing those cells with PCR techniques, FISH techniques, or cytogenetic techniques. Perhaps even before fetal cell rescue becomes routinely useful, PCR techniques are likely to be useful for identifying uniparental disomy in prenatal diagnosis specimens. Two common scenarios for using this approach would include (1) an ostensibly normal fetal karyotype in the presence of abnormal fetal ultrasound findings; and (2) the presence of an ostensibly balanced fetal chromosome rearrangement (which, in approximately 10 percent of cases, leads to an adverse outcome).

New Treatment

Treating genetic disorders requires knowing the precise disturbance at the biochemical level, the molecular (DNA) level, or both. There are five general types of treatment of genetic disorders: (1) making up for a deficient metabolic product by *supplying* that product directly (e.g., vitamin B12) or driving an alternative reaction by supplying a critical, rate-limiting cofactor (e.g., pyridoxine-sensitive homocystinuria); (2) *avoiding* substrates (e.g., drugs, nutrients) that would have toxic effects (e.g., furadantoin in G-6-PD deficiency); (3) *decreasing* an excessive amount of a metabolic product (e.g., a phenylalanine-poor diet in phenylketonuria); (4) *replacing* an absent or functionally deficient *gene product* (e.g., Factor VIII in Hemophilia A, glucocerebrosidase in Gaucher disease); and (5) replacing the absent or functionally deficient *gene*.

The last two types of genetic treatment have become realistic as a result of the HGP and related research. As we identify and clone each human gene, we can then use them to make large amounts of the respective gene products to permit gene-product replacement therapy. An alternative is to engineer bacterial or cultured tissue cells (or even cell-free systems using PCR techniques) to produce the genes themselves in sufficient quantity for insertion into intact tissues in the affected person. Gene-replacement therapy already appears to be feasible for both types of disorder (Anderson, 1992).

Another treatment approach involves *prevention*. Preimplantation genetics involves identifying a mutant gene in germ cells (e.g., polar body biopsy) or very early embryos. Alternatively, germ cells or very early embryos can be identified that are *free of the mutation* in question. Thus, embryos resulting from in vitro fertilization and shown to be free of a mutation at a specific locus can be implanted in the womb for further natural development.

Strategies for Clinician Genetic Education

Techniques

Although this presentation is directed at the clinician already in practice, it is obvious that another way to approach educating clinicians about medical genetics is at the original source, medical school. Recent surveys (Riccardi & Schmickel, 1988) have indicated a wide variation in medical school genetic teaching, both because the total number of teaching hours varies greatly and because the responsibility for teaching genetics falls to several different departments, including biochemistry, genetics, and pediatrics. Although it is doubtful that more teaching time labeled as "genetics" will be forthcoming, certainly there will be more genetics taught. An increase in the number of departments of genetics in medical schools is probably the key to improving teaching at that level, whether or not the genetics department assumes sole responsibility for the teaching effort. The HGP can and should provide impetus to that end.

Medical specialty boards represent a unique opportunity to influence burgeoning clinicians about the importance of medical, that is, clinical, genetics. Presently, the emphasis is minor and highly variable. The organizers of the HGP might well consider providing for a specific liaison person to work with the specialty boards (e.g., pediatrics, obstetrics, oncology) to effect this approach to capitalizing on the proceeds of the project. It remains to be seen whether the establishment of a program for board certification of medical geneticists and the newly formed American College of Medical Genetics will enhance this opportunity.

But, back to the practicing clinician. If we agree that a good grasp of genetics is increasingly critical in the work of modern clinicians, how are we to go about educating them? There are three ways of reaching clinicians: at the bedside, through case reports, and by topics.

Bedside (Consultation)

The bedside remains a potent setting for teaching. Geneticists who provide consultation services should communicate to the referring clinician both the details relevant to the proband (or consultand) and the generalizations that can be applied to future patients. In short, every genetics consultation interaction must involve a specific effort by the geneticist to generalize the principles derived from the individual case; in other words, to teach.

Case Reports

Some cases may be so instructive (e.g., cystic fibrosis resulting from uniparental isodisomy) that written case reports and presentations at clinical conferences and departmental grand rounds are obligatory. This is not a new insight. What might be new, however, is the obligation of the clinical geneticist to ensure that such presentations benefit general clinicians.

Topical

Clinical geneticists who provide written manuscripts, oral presentations, or both, must increase their efforts to provide such resources directly to clinicians in various types of summary forms that go beyond the bedside and the case reports. The focus may be on a particular disease (e.g., NF-1) or sets of diseases (e.g., neurocutaneous disorders) or on technologies (e.g., PCR, FISH). The format may be written articles or lectures. This has been done in the past, but geneticists must make a deliberate effort to collaborate with publishers, editors, directors of continuing medical education programs, and other resources to ensure that clinicians are being reached.

The Teachers

Individuals

Who should be responsible for these teaching efforts? Scientists with a clinical bent can be especially useful for reaching both medium-sized and large audiences; for example, through lectures at major medical meetings (e.g., American Academy of Pediatrics). Clinical geneticists, particularly those with a keen appreciation of the molecular biology principles and facts, can and must make similar presentations, as well as presentations to smaller groups; for example, in local hospitals.

Medical genetics has defined and developed a relatively new profession—that currently referred to as "genetic counselors," in the past also known as "genetic associates." My preference for the latter designation respects the fact that these Masters Degree specialists often devote themselves to tasks other than genetic counseling. These professionals play increasingly important roles in developing, coordinating and implementing genetic education programs; they are a major resource for education.

Organizations

Only a handful of medical geneticists and genetic counselors are in private practice. The vast majority function under the aegis of a larger organization.

Medical Schools and Other Institutions of Higher Education. These organizations, particularly those that have received substantial funding for participation in the HGP at the research level, have a special obligation to meet the educational needs outlined here. Increasingly, funding for research should require specific teaching efforts directed at the clinician. The argument for presuming this obligation is that the HGP has been presented to the citizenry as an opportunity for *all* of them to capitalize on. And the only way to effect this intention is for the main users of the information—namely, clinicians—to be versed in both the broad principles and specific details derived from the project.

Education Firms. Many other organizations focus on education, whether from a profit motive (e.g., publishers, videotape producers) or as a nonprofit organization (e.g., Biological Sciences Curriculum Study, Colorado Springs, CO). It is feasible and, in my opinion, necessary to encourage both the establishment of more such organizations and their exploitation on behalf of the HGP. A coordinated series of programs should be developed for the widespread, cost-effective teaching of medical genetics to clinicians.

Specific Teaching Mechanisms

In designing teaching programs, six general considerations should be taken into account. Moreover, continuing medical education programs directed at primary-care and secondary-care clinicians have not been fully exploited. Providing CME credits as part of the various approaches listed below is an obvious, perhaps necessary, way to enhance the prospects of medical genetics education efforts.

Subscription Mailings

Printed. Newsletters and quarterly journals directed at non-geneticists are a very effective means for increasing knowledge about medical genetics. Subsidies to facilitate low subscription rates could be provided from federal government research funding sources, biotechnology corporations, nonprofit foundations, and private philanthropy.

Audio Recordings and Video Recordings. This popular means of continuing medical education has not been utilized at all for teaching medical genetics, even though other branches of medicine have shown it to be both effective and affordable.

Interactive Computer Programs. The use of rapid microprocessors combined with CD-ROM technology and graphic presentation programs has been virtually ignored for teaching medical genetics.

Non-subscription Mailings

Printed materials, recordings, and computer aids can also be adapted to non-subscription mailing techniques. One-time purchases or free items (subsidized as noted above) could be highly effective, especially if combined with the prospect of obtaining continuing medical education credits.

Journal Articles, Books, and Chapters

The emphasis here is on journal articles in publications that ordinarily do not focus on genetics and articles that respect the limited genetic knowledge of clinicians. Rather than the geneticists continuing to write to and for themselves, we need a concerted effort to write for clinicians in general.

Symposia, Seminars and Workshops

Stand-alone presentations focusing on genetics may be a long-term goal, but, presently it is difficult to induce clinicians to give up large blocks of time to focus on genetics. A first step would be to incorporate elements of genetic education into broader program formats. For example, one might focus on having such programs as part of annual meetings of major specialty and subspecialty professional groups.

Lectures

Lectures as part of continuing programs such as departmental grand rounds are an excellent way to reach a "captive audience." Waiting passively for the invitation will not work, however. Rather, there should be a concerted, coordinated effort to ensure that medical genetics lectures are regularly given with the specific intent of covering the consequences and meaning of the HGP and similar projects.

Consultations

As noted already, the bedside or clinic consultation is a very effective way to teach general principles. However, the medical geneticist may need occasional reminders to address the broader long-term teaching goals.

Content of Clinician Genetic Education Courses and Materials

These teaching efforts could focus on a variety of aspects of the new genetics. There would be no need to deal with them all at once, although this might be done in the occasional symposium or workshop devoted to this range of topics.

Clinical

Clinicians are, after all, clinicians, and making the subject matter clinically relevant is key. It can be done relatively easily: clinical practice presently requires a knowledge of genetics; the current discussion is merely a setting for making that statement experientially.

Pathogenesis/Clinical Correlations

Knowledge of the basic genetic defect (mutation) increasingly provides information about the clinical progression of a disorder. Cystic fibrosis, NF-1, NF-2, sickle cell anemia, the Li-Fraumeni syndrome, the aniridia-Wilms tumor complex, and the Prader-Willi syndrome, are but a few examples among heritable genetic disorders. Chronic myelogenous leukemia, colon cancer, neurofibrosarcomas, and many other malignancies are examples among the acquired (somatic) genetic disorders. As the relation between genetic aberrations and clinical consequences becomes increasingly clear, particularly if it improves prognosis and therapy, clinicians will develop an appetite for this type of knowledge. Again, lessons learned from the development of coordinated interactions of infectious-disease specialists and clinicians (e.g., use of vaccines, respect for a wide array of microbes, and highly specific therapies) are relevant to the genetic model being considered here.

Forensic

The forensic application of knowledge of the human genome is likely to be of interest to many clinicians, including issues of nonpaternity, rape, and child abuse.

Basic Research

Finally, although basic research may not capture the attention of clinicians for long, there are reasons to include it in educational programs. First, clinicians are graduates of programs that emphasize (and select for) intellectual curiosity. Many clinicians simply will want to have some idea about the underpinnings of the clinical and pathogenetic consequences of genetic disorders. Second, there is the matter of reinforcing the notion of constant progress. Even if the details are not retained, many clinicians might well be impressed by the momentum and direction of the research, further instilling a conviction about the relevance of newly acquired knowledge about genetic disease.

References

Anderson W. F. (1992) Human gene therapy. *Science*, 256:808–13.

Caskey C. T., Pizzuti A., Fu Y-H, et al. (1992) Triplet repeat mutations in human disease. *Science*, 256:784–89.

Devilee P., Van den Broek M., Mannens M., et al. (1991) Differences in patterns of allelic loss between two common types of adult cancer, breast and colon carcinoma, and Wilms' tumor of childhood. *International Journal of Cancer*, 47:817–21.

Engel E., DeLozier-Blanchet C. D. (1991) Uniparental disomy, isodisomy, and imprinting: Probable effects in man and strategies for their detection. *American Journal of Medicine Genetics*, 40:432–39.

Ferguson-Smith A. C., Reik W., Surani M. A. (1990) Genomic imprinting and cancer. *Cancer Surveys*, 9:487–503.

Hackerman N. (1992) Science education: Who needs it? *Science*, 256:157.

Hall J. G. (1990) Genomic imprinting: Review and relevance to human diseases. *American Journal of Human Genetics*, 46:857–73.

Hall J. G. (1992) Genomic imprinting and its clinical implications. *New England Journal of Medicine*, 326:827–28.

Heutink P., van der May A. G. L., Sandkuijl L. A., et al. (1992) A gene subject to genomic imprinting and responsible for hereditary paragangliomas maps to chromosome 11q23-qter. *Human Molecular Genetics*, 1:7–10.

Hulten M. A., Gould C. P., Goldman A. S. H., Waters J. J. (1991) Chromosome in situ suppression hybridisation in clinical cytogenetics. *Journal of Medical Genetics*, 28:577-82.

Lupski J. R., Wise C. A., Kuwano A., et al. (1992) Gene dosage is a mechanism for Charcot-Marie-Tooth disease type 1A. *Nature Genetics*, 1:29-33.

Mahadevan M., Tsifidis C., Sabourin L., et al. (1992) Myotonic dystrophy mutation: An unstable CTG repeat in the 3' untranslated region of the gene. *Science*, 255:1253-55.

Marshall C. J. (1991) Tumor suppressor genes. *Cell*, 64:313-26.

Risch N.J., Devlin B. (1992) On the probability of matching DNA fingerprints. *Science*, 255:717-20.

Rousseau F., Heitz D., Biancalana V., et al. (1991) Direct diagnosis by DNA analysis of the Fragile X syndrome of mental retardation. *New England Journal of Medicine*, 325:1673-81.

Riccardi V. M., Schmickel R. D. (1988) Human genetics as a component of medical school curricula: A report to the American Society of Human Genetics. *American Journal of Human Genetics*, 42:639-43.

Sidransky D., von Eschenbach A., Tsai Y. C., et al. (1991) Identification of p53 gene mutations in bladder cancers and urine samples. *Science*, 252:706-709.

Sidransky D., Tokino T., Hamilton S. R. (1992) Identification of ras oncogene mutations in the stool of patients with curable colorectal tumors. *Science*, 256:102-105.

Zhang Y., Tycko B. (1992) Monoallelic expression of the human H19 gene. *Nature Genetics*, 1:40-44.

Three

Medicine, Gene Therapy, and Society

William J. Polvino and W. French Anderson

The therapeutic armamentarium for the treatment of diseases encompasses many treatment modalities. Counseling, dietary modification, and various forms of physical therapies can be employed in the treatment or prevention of ailments. A vast compendium of chemical agents, drugs, are available, as well as surgical or radiation techniques that have been developed. Despite the extent of medical treatments at our disposal, frequently patients are left suffering, in need of improved therapy. A fundamental difficulty is often encountered: we find ourselves able to treat the manifestations of a disease but not its source.

Human gene therapy is a potentially powerful new class of therapeutics. Gene therapy is the intentional introduction of exogenous genetic material into a patient (or the patient's cells) to achieve a therapeutic goal. In contrast, the term "gene marking" denotes the introduction of genetic material from which no direct therapeutic benefit is anticipated.

The potential demand for gene therapy is real. Many diseases remain inadequately treated and are the source of morbidity and mortality. It is estimated that single gene defects are present in 10 out of every 1000 live births (Carter, 1977). Furthermore, there may be an element of genetic contribution to nearly all human diseases (Childs, 1988). If improvements in gene therapy prove that it is safe and effective, resources to deliver treatment may be overwhelmed by demand. A situation similar to organ transplantation could result in which societal value judgments may enter into decisions regarding allocation of a limited resource (Walters, 1986; Ramsey, 1970). The problem is magnified if one considers the global community and the disparities in access to health care already present.

The access of an individual to an effective gene therapy may in the future depend on the ability to pay for that treatment or, more importantly, the willingness of medical insurers to reimburse for such therapy. An analogous situation already exists for bone marrow transplant technology, for which insurers make difficult decisions regarding the appropriate indications for such treatment. In such a market, gene therapy will no doubt be required to prove it is both medically and economically sound.

The genetic material introduced via human gene therapy techniques is generally intended to provide a "blueprint" for the production of a therapeutic protein. Thus, human gene therapy may be considered a pharmacologic treatment in which the patient's body is provided the means to manufacture a helpful protein. As such, this technology may ultimately allow patients to produce naturally-occurring proteins with beneficial effects under circumstances in which the body would not normally produce the desired quantities. One of the key research problems is to identify the gene responsible for producing the protein of interest.

Molecular Basis of Gene Therapy

The techniques to manipulate DNA in the laboratory have allowed contemplation of "genetic surgery." The discovery of enzymes known as restriction endonucleases permit scientists to cut long strands of DNA at precise locations. These segments of DNA can then be separated and spliced together in desired arrangements. Small circular DNA structures, plasmids, accept these engineered DNA fragments and allow them to be replicated in the laboratory (i.e., "cloned"). In this way, normal human genes have been identified and cloned; some of these may be used for gene therapy upon introduction into the desired "target" cells. A variety of techniques have been employed to introduce genes into cells, the simplest of which is to physically inject the DNA into target cells. Physical injection is labor-intensive and quite inefficient for most applications. A more practical approach is to utilize naturally occurring viruses, retroviruses, which inject foreign genes into cells as part of their natural life cycles.[1] These viruses can be engineered, using cutting and splicing techniques, to destroy their ability to replicate and to use them as "vectors" to carry the desired gene(s) into the target cell. This is the method currently employed for most gene therapy protocols.

Human Gene Therapy

Human gene therapy was conceived in the 1960s; in the early 1970s, the first successful DNA splicing experiments were performed. The prospect of genuine therapy gained momentum as molecular understanding of human disease grew and as additional experiments proved that foreign genes were able to function inside host cells.

The initial enthusiasm was met with controversy, though, following an unauthorized experiment involving two patients with beta-thalassemia (Sun, 1981). The outcome was official censure of the investigator and a growing sentiment that human gene therapy experimentation called for thoughtful deliberation of its scientific and ethical merits. Subsequent initiation of gene marking/gene therapy studies in the United States required approval of the National Institutes of Health's (NIH's) Recombinant DNA Advisory Committee (RAC) and the Human Gene Therapy Subcommittee (HGTSC) of the RAC. In addition, approval by the Food and Drug Administration (FDA) and the local institutional review board was required.

The first clinical protocol to receive approval (in 1989) through this extensive review was a study at the NIH with patients with terminal malignant melanoma. A protocol had been underway since 1986, investigating the treatment of cancer patients with immune cells grown from their tumor biopsies, tumor-infiltrating lymphocytes (TIL). These cells were isolated from the biopsy and grown in culture in the presence of hormones which caused them to multiply. The cells were then reinfused into the patients in an effort to provide stimulated immune cells to attack the remaining cancer cells. Approximately 35–40 percent of the patients showed responses to the TIL therapy; in some cases, complete remissions were observed. It was not possible, however, to predict which patients would respond to the treatment, nor was it possible to explain why the treatment would work in some patients but not others. The gene marking experiment, while not intended to provide a therapeutic gene, allowed a proportion of the cells to be genetically labeled in an effort to identify subsets of TIL cells most effective in attacking tumor cells. The study was designed to help explain the reasons for the unpredictable clinical responses and consequently allow for refinement of TIL therapy.

The results of the study showed that the marked TILs could be identified in the patient's blood, as well as in tumor biopsies, for up to three months following treatment (Rosenberg et al., 1990). In addition, there were no side effects attributable to the gene transfer process.

The first actual human gene *therapy* proposal which was approved and carried out was for the treatment of adenosine deaminase (ADA)-deficient severe combined immunodeficiency disease (SCID). Children with ADA-deficient SCID suffer from recurrent infections, and often die in childhood as a result of their weakened immune system. This initial gene therapy study proposed to introduce the gene for ADA into patients' white blood cells. The protocol called for periodic removal of blood from the patient; the blood cells would be separated, with the red blood cells returned to the patient and the defective white blood cells grown in culture in a laboratory. The patient's cells would be treated with an engineered retroviral vector which could introduce the gene for ADA. The cells would then be reinfused into the patient. The objective of the study was to show that introduction of the functional ADA gene into the patient's white blood cells would cause no harm and would improve the ability of the defective white blood cells to fight infection.

The protocol was reviewed in total by six regulatory bodies over a period of seven months. The review of the gene therapy protocol was considered to be the most extensive review of a clinical protocol ever conducted.[2] The protocol was initiated on September 14, 1990. To date, two patients have been treated in the study.

The first patient to receive ADA gene therapy was a four-year-old girl who received gene-corrected white blood cells once every one to two months for 10.5 months. The level of ADA detectable in her circulating white blood cells was initially less than 1 percent of the normal level. With treatments, this level rose to 25 percent of the normal value and showed no significant fall during an intentional 6.5 month interval without retreatment. More importantly, the patient was able to demonstrate immune responses against foreign antigens, such as vaccines, to which she was exposed. The patient has suffered no significant ill effects as a result of receiving the gene-corrected white blood cells and is now able to attend school. A second patient, a nine-year-old girl, has begun to receive treatments, and again has shown no signs of ill effects from the therapy. Both patients continue to be monitored for therapeutic effects as well as to be evaluated for possible adverse reactions.

Present Status of Human Gene Therapy

The initial results of the ADA gene therapy protocol are promising, however the treatment technique corrects the genetic defect in a population of predominantly mature white blood cells. It is thought that different mature white blood cells are able to mount an immune response against different foreign antigens. The gene therapy treatments insert the ADA gene into a fraction of the cells and as such may strengthen the immune capabilities of some cells, but not others. As a result, "holes" may be left in the immune "repertoire" of the patient (Anderson, 1992) and the patient may remain susceptible to some infections. A revised ADA gene therapy protocol has been proposed to attempt treatment of a more immature population of circulating white blood cells in an effort to correct progenitor cells with the capacity to give rise to multiple mature white blood cells. The revised protocol has received approval from the Recombinant DNA Advisory Committee and the FDA. Similar protocols to investigate the treatment of SCID are underway in Milan, Italy, and the Netherlands (Anderson, 1992).

The initial gene-marking work in melanoma patients has been expanded to use gene therapy in an attempt to further enhance the body's immune capacity to fight cancer cells. Clinical studies are investigating the potential efficacy of immune cells modified with genes encoding biologically active proteins such as tumor necrosis factor (TNF) or interleukin-2 (IL-2). The gene for TNF has been inserted into TIL cells and the modified cells infused into patients. TNF displays potent anticancer effects in mice; however the high doses required are toxic to humans. TIL cells are able to localize to the site of tumor deposits and, therefore, gene-modified TIL cells may be able to provide high levels of TNF locally at the tumor site without exposing the body to toxic levels. In separate studies, the gene for either TNF or IL-2 is inserted into the tumor cells themselves and the modified tumor cells injected into the patient. These modified tumor cells may trigger a more vigorous immune attack from the patient's white blood cells. A study has also been initiated at the St. Jude Children's Research Hospital to investigate IL-2 gene therapy in the treatment of neuroblastoma.

Gene-marking experiments similar to the initial TIL-marking study in melanoma patients are underway at the University of Pittsburgh, UCLA, and in Lyon, France.

Gene-marking techniques are being investigated to analyze the biology of cancer relapse following bone marrow transplantation for childhood acute myelogenous leukemia[3] and neuroblastoma,[4] as well as for adult leukemias.[5,6] A patient undergoing treatment has bone marrow removed prior to treatment. The patient then receives lethal doses of chemotherapy to eliminate cancer cells and the bone marrow is then reinfused to rescue the patient. If the cancer recurs following such treatment, it is unclear whether the cancer cells were remaining in the patient's body and/or if they were present in the reinfused bone marrow. By genetically marking the bone marrow cells, the source of the relapsing cancer cells may be identified. Other protocols are investigating bone marrow transplantation and the physiology of cancer relapse in multiple myeloma and breast cancer. Studies have also been approved to investigate the fate of liver cells which have been marked and infused into patients with acute hepatic failure.[7]

A clinical gene therapy study is underway to investigate the safety and efficacy of infusing liver cells modified to express the low density lipoprotein receptor into patients with a congenital lack of these receptors: an often lethal condition known as familial hypercholesterolemia.[8] An additional gene therapy protocol initiated in China addresses the potential for treatment of hemophilia B with cells genetically modified to secrete the missing clotting factor, Factor IX.[9]

In evaluating this extensive list of new clinical studies, a few points are noteworthy. First, the growth in number of clinical studies is significant. This reflects a desire on the part of the medical community to investigate the potential applications of this technique. Second, the majority of the studies involve the ex vivo manipulation of cells. This methodology provides that cells are removed from patients, genetically altered in the laboratory, and reinfused into patients, thus providing the opportunity to characterize the manipulated cells prior to reintroduction into patients. The requirement to perform genetic manipulations outside of the patient's body is, however, a barrier to the development of human gene therapy, since it increases the complexity of the treatment compared to more conventional modalities.

Two protocols have been approved in which gene therapy vectors will be introduced directly into the patient's body. In the first, investigators at the University of Michigan have injected a gene therapy vector into tumor deposits of malignant melanoma.[10] The vector contains information to express a cell surface protein (histocompatibility antigen) which if produced by the tumor cells could lead to destruction of the melanoma by enhancement of the body's immune attack upon the cells. The second study, to be performed at the NIH, uses gene therapy to introduce the gene for a viral enzyme (herpes simplex thymidine kinase) into brain tumors.[11] If the tumor cells produce the viral enzyme, they will become susceptible to killing by the antiviral drug, gancyclovir. The technique should selectively destroy tumor cells, since the rapidly dividing brain tumor cells will preferentially incorporate the vector and express the protein, while the normal brain cells (which are largely nondividing) should not.

Gene therapy technology is also being applied in efforts to treat or prevent acquired immunodeficiency syndrome (AIDS). In one study, white blood cells treated in the laboratory are infused back into patients with AIDS in an attempt to enhance the immune attack on the AIDS virus in a fashion analogous to TIL therapy for melanoma.[12] A gene therapy vector is used to insert the herpes simplex thymidine kinase gene into the cells. As such, the treatment may be terminated, if desired, by infusing gancyclovir, thus selectively destroying the manipulated cells. Use of such a "suicide vector," while not directly beneficial to the patient, enhances the safety of the treatment by enabling the cellular therapy to be terminated if necessary. The second investigation employs gene therapy to produce an experimental AIDS immunotherapeutic, a treatment designed not to attack the AIDS virus, per se, but rather to strengthen the body's natural immune defenses to fight the disease more effectively. In this study, gene therapy will be used to engineer cells to produce proteins from the AIDS virus to stimulate the body's immune attack.

Potential Applications of Human Gene Therapy

Human gene therapy has prompted diverse investigation and consequent scientific creativity in hypothesizing potential applications, the actualization of which will depend, in large part, on the results of the initial trials, technologic developments, available resources, and societal choices. The variety of potential therapies is, at times, surprising even to those familiar with the technology.

There are several homozygous recessive diseases which are targets for gene therapy, potentially within this decade. Lesch-Nyhan syndrome, alpha-1-antitrypsin deficiency, cystic fibrosis, hemophilia A and B, Gaucher disease, beta-thalassemia, sickle cell anemia, and Duchenne's muscular dystrophy are genetic diseases which extract heavy tolls in suffering and for which the necessary genes have been identified.[13] Proposed clinical studies for some of these diseases are already underway.

The development of clinical protocols for additional homozygous recessive genetic illnesses is certain. However, the potential reach of gene therapy applications is not limited to the "classic" inborn genetic diseases.

A number of protocols have already been proposed using gene therapy in an attempt to treat cancer (see above). Current chemotherapeutic treatment of many cancers involves administering toxic drugs which are able to kill cancerous cells more effectively than normal cells but, unfortunately, still extract a toll on normally functioning cells. The result of this non-specificity is toxicity to the patient. The effect is a reduction in blood elements (including infection-fighting white blood cells) to dangerously low levels, which can be fatal when the chemotherapy kills too many normal bone marrow cells. A strategy has been envisaged to treat normal bone marrow cells prior to chemotherapy by inserting the gene for multiple drug resistance (MDR). The treatment could make bone marrow cells more resistant to toxic effects from subsequent chemotherapy, allowing higher doses of drugs to be administered. The probability for successful treatment of the cancer may thus be increased.

Alternative approaches to treating cancer include introducing genes for cellular hormones such as IL-2 or gamma interferon to convert cancerous cells into benign cells (Tremisis and Bich-Thuy, 1991; Nadkarni, Datar, and Rao, 1991) or to prompt an immune attack upon malignant cells. Additionally, the cancer process is now believed to be due, in part, to the loss of normal cellular proteins—the absence of which leads to malignancy and spread. Gene therapy may provide a means to restore "normalcy" to these aberrant cells. A growing number of genes, including the p53 gene and the retinoblastoma gene, have demonstrated the ability to suppress cellular changes leading to the malignant phenotype.[14] In addition, cellular communication channels, known as gap junctions, are coded for by genes and may prove of therapeutic benefit in restoring normal communication links in malignant cells, reverting them to a benign state. As such, cancer may be thought of as an acquired genetic disorder and applications of gene therapy may become avenues of treatment. Gene therapy vectors may also be potentially used to kill cancer cells by inactivating proteins peculiar to cancer cells which are necessary for their survival or by producing a toxin once taken up by the cancer cell.

The treatment of infectious diseases, particularly AIDS, has become an area of active gene therapy investigation (Jolly, 1991). In addition to the immunotherapeutic cell therapy studies in AIDS patients (described above), researchers are investigating the use of gene therapy to block infection by the secretion of "dummy receptors" into the blood stream which bind the virus until it can be eliminated from the body (Morgan et al., 1990). Other approaches employ the concept of "in vitro immunization" in which uninfected cells are treated with genes designed to combat a virus attempting to gain entry into the cell (Faraji-Shadan, Stubbs, and Bowman, 1990). Genes have been designed to generate ribozymes, molecules of RNA which possess the ability to enzymatically cleave specific segments of DNA. Such ribozymes may provide a treatment strategy when engineered to disrupt DNA necessary for propagation of the AIDS virus.

Gene therapy has been employed to secrete clot-dissolving proteins into the blood in an effort, ultimately, to treat or prevent recurrent coronary artery disease, in which formation of blood clots in the narrowed arteries may lead to angina or heart attacks by obstructing blood flow. The use of genetically modified cells to coat intravascular stents (which prop open narrow arteries) have been investigated with the objective of preventing the recurrent narrowing, restenosis, of the artery (Dichek et al., 1989). Direct administration of gene therapy vectors to cells lining arteries during catheterization procedures may provide a convenient means to administer such treatments. This methodology has been studied in animals with some preliminary success.

Coronary artery disease may also one day be treated by gene therapy with angiogenesis factor genes, genes designed to promote the growth of new blood vessels, to provide additional blood flow to areas which are threatened by limited perfusion through narrowed vessels.

Neurologic disorders had been thought an area for which gene therapy would be difficult, due to the peculiarities of neuronal tissues. Effective incorporation of gene therapy vectors often requires active growth and division of the target cells; mature nerve cells generally do not divide. The herpes virus family, however, is able to infect neurons; scientists have recently developed gene therapy vectors using modified herpes viruses (Geller et al., 1990; Freese and Geller, 1991). Such vectors may prove useful in providing therapeutic proteins to treat neurologic disease. For example, the gene for the enzyme tyrosine hydroxylase has been cloned and may be applied in the treatment of Parkinson's disease, a disorder thought due to deficiency of the neurotransmitter dopamine. Tyrosine hydroxylase is important in the production of dopamine; gene therapy with the enzyme may assist in correcting the deficiency. Other scientists are investigating engraving genetically modified cells into nervous tissue (Gage et al., 1990).

Applications of gene therapy have, in fact, been conceived for a wide array of disorders including kidney stones (Lung, Cornelius and Peck, 1991) and arthritis.—the latter from the observation that cells lining joint spaces are capable of incorporating retroviral vectors (Bandara et al., 1992). Gene therapy may be viewed as a pharmacologic means to provide sustained delivery of a therapeutic protein. As such, treatments for common endocrinologic maladies such as diabetes mellitus and osteoporosis have been proposed.

There are limits, however, to the existing methods. The initial clinical study for the treatment of ADA-deficient SCID illustrates the present technologic difficulties with human gene therapy. To treat one child, months of effort and extensive analysis were required to produce clinical-grade treatment materials; the child was brought to the clinical center twice every month, once to have blood cells removed and once to receive the reinfusion of modified cells. Evaluation and monitoring of the child continues on an indefinite basis; extensive counseling and administrative follow-up are necessary. These steps are important to ensure the safety of the patients in the first study, given the novel nature of gene therapy. It would, however, be difficult to envisage that gene therapy will be applied to a wide range of disorders unless the method could be demonstrated to be safe, practical, and not prohibitively expensive. Notwithstanding, there may remain a place for gene therapy using existing technology in the treatment of those illnesses, such as ADA-deficient SCID, for which treatment options are limited.

Technologic Issues

At present the methodology for clinical gene therapy studies is labor-intensive, inefficient, and costly. The laboratory techniques of molecular biology continue to be explored as this methodology is an integral component of much scientific research. This continued research provides a foundation from which refinements of technique may be developed. Ultimately these advancements in laboratory technology may allow improvement in the methodology for clinical administration of gene therapy.

Efforts are underway to generate vectors which may be directly applied to subjects, such as by inhalational aerosol (Rosenfeld et al., 1992) or injection, avoiding the difficulties with ex vivo manipulation of cellular cultures. Non-viral means of genetic delivery, such as by proteoliposomes, are being investigated. The ability to deliver functional genes precisely to replace defective genes by gene targeting (Capecchi, 1989) could prove to be an advance for both the safety and the efficacy of gene therapy.

A further technologic goal of gene therapy is to introduce therapeutic genes into cells which have the capacity to replicate throughout the life of patients. The extended life span of such cells could provide a means to extend the therapeutic benefit from a given treatment with the desired gene. "Stem cells" (Golde, 1991) are present in the bone marrow and possess the ability for replication and differentiation into the various lineages of blood cells. These cells, while not yet fully characterized, are believed to possess a life-long replicative capacity. As the bone marrow is relatively accessible by needle biopsy, these cells are attractive targets for gene therapy (Kantoff, Freeman, and Anderson, 1988).

For the immediate future, gene therapy remains a methodologic challenge which limits its utility in potential applications and accessibility to patients. It is a field, however, which continues to evolve; the role of gene therapy in medical practice will be dependent upon this evolution. For example, it is conceivable that cystic fibrosis may be treated by periodic, aerosolized, gene transfer treatments.

Regulatory Issues

At present any gene therapy study utilizing federal funding is required to be reviewed and approved by the Recombinant DNA Advisory Committee (RAC) and by the director of the National Institutes of Health. These steps are in addition to the submission of the protocol for standard clinical review by the local institutional review board and institutional biosafety committee (Areen and King, 1990). Protection of human subjects in the United States is further regulated by federal restrictions[15] via the FDA. The study protocol and materials to be utilized must be approved by the FDA for studies conducted in the United States, as for any investigational drug or medical product.

Two points are noteworthy in the review process. First, non–NIH-funded studies, such as corporate studies, are not obligated to obtain approval from the RAC. However, corporate sponsors may voluntarily submit to the RAC for review and are encouraged to do so. For reasons of liability, additional review may be highly advisable in such a novel investigational area (Palmer, 1991; Mackler, 1990). Failure to do so at an early stage in development may be viewed as a departure from the customary review process and expose a sponsor to extensive liability. Second, regulatory requirements vary greatly among countries. The NIH and the FDA are not involved in oversight of studies conducted outside of the United States. The principles of independent review and protection of human subjects are, however, adhered to by the international community; the procedures vary by which individual countries ensure that these principles are observed.

Regulatory review serves an important purpose. It provides an objective means by which the safety of human subjects can be reasonably assured while allowing technology to advance. The FDA evaluates gene therapy proposals to ensure that both the product to be employed and the process by which the product was manufactured meet acceptable standards (Epstein, 1991). The proposal is evaluated in terms of its safety and in terms of the probability that the product, process, and/or protocol will perform as intended. The field of gene therapy is a new area for regulatory agencies and will require evolving guidelines to assure that these goals are achieved. To this end, both the FDA[16] and RAC[17] have issued "Points to Consider" documents to serve as guidelines for the development of gene therapy proposals. The present regulatory process for gene therapy studies is extensive, as witnessed by the protracted debate prior to the first gene therapy study (Carmen, 1992; Roberts, 1989). Such extensive review will not always be necessary as more knowledge is acquired in the field and review committees are better able to objectively evaluate proposed studies.

A technology which raises ethical concerns, such as human gene therapy, may be subjected to a tendency to impose increased regulatory constraints.[18] For the field of gene therapy, this reaction could be damaging. When faced with the prospect of excessive regulatory constraints, scientists and investors may be discouraged from pursuing the area. Potential benefits from the technology may go unrealized. The negative impact of excessive regulation requires consideration. The increased restrictions recently placed on molecular biologists in Germany has influenced scientific investigation, generating fears that Germany will be disadvantaged in its ability to attract and retain promising scientists (Kahn, 1992). Widespread restriction could similarly hamper development and discourage investigation in the field of human gene therapy.

The need for objective review of medical treatments is evident. Prior to the implementation of FDA requirements, unproven elixirs were marketed for medicinal purposes based on testimonial evidence. These so-called "medications" were in certain instances clearly dangerous (Gelling and Cannon, 1938; "Deaths" [editorial], 1937). The existing regulations for drug development were designed to ensure that medical treatments are appropriately safe and effective for their intended purposes. A therapeutic from a novel field of investigation, such as human gene therapy, merits more thorough evaluation than, for example, a new drug which has been developed from a field in which extensive experience is available. A flexible approach to the field of gene therapy allows regulatory practices to evolve as experience and technology develop.

Financial Considerations

Presently, gene therapy is expensive. The number of scientists involved in treating ADA-deficient SCID, for example, exceeds the number of afflicted patients. Added to the personnel costs are the costs of research and development, quality control, clinical, monitoring, regulatory, and administrative expenses. Human gene therapy studies require research subsidy from either governmental or private (e.g., corporate) sponsors. If gene therapy does prove to be an effective treatment for otherwise devastating illnesses, a high treatment cost may be competitive against the "conventional" treatment costs and societal costs associated with morbidity and mortality.

The success of the initial studies with gene therapy and the technologic developments which follow will dictate the mode of administration of the therapy, the frequency of the treatments, the diseases to be treated, and the cost of a course of therapy.

Estimation of the target population for all forms of gene therapy is presently error-prone, largely due to the limited clinical experience with such treatment. The ultimate size of the target population for a given therapeutic application is dependent upon the prevalence of the disease under consideration and assumptions regarding the anticipated safety and efficacy profile of the therapeutic, derived from experience in well-controlled clinical studies. It can be projected that a treatment which demonstrates significant efficacy with few adverse experiences (and thus a favorable benefit-to-risk ratio) may be applied to a large segment of the patient population, while a treatment with a less favorable profile would be reserved for treatment of only the most severely afflicted patients, who may have failed other, more conventional, therapies.

Similarly, projection of the cost of treatment with gene therapy is problematic. Each specific indication must be considered separately with assessment of the costs for production and requirements for support of the product to ensure availability to patients. Additionally, assumptions are necessary to estimate the potential target population for the product as well as the ability for the new treatment to "penetrate" into this market. "Penetration" is, in turn, dependent upon the nature of the disease, the presumed willingness of patients to try (and physicians to prescribe) the new treatment, availability and adequacy of existing therapies, advantages and disadvantages of the new treatment in comparison to existing options, presumed dosing regimen of the gene therapy, and the estimated price which will be charged per unit of treatment. Such estimations allow for projection of the overall net profit (or loss) from development of the treatment.

The competitiveness of gene therapy in the market is thus highly dependent upon the adequacy of available treatments versus the projected advantages of the specific gene therapy application, as well as the costs of production. As stated previously, current treatments in many disease categories fall short in their ability to effectively treat disease and rarely offer a "cure." Gene therapy may offer significant, competitive advantages due to the qualitatively different mechanism of therapy. With continued development, gene therapy as a treatment class may become available in a context similar to other, more conventional, pharmaceutical options for the prescribing physician.

The Human Genome Project

Analysis of the human genome in its entirety will help provide the information by which new gene therapies can be developed. An enhanced understanding of human physiology and pathophysiology can be gained. Understanding disease at the molecular level may add to our ability to diagnose and treat diseases more accurately and earlier in their course (Green and Waterston, 1991). The limitations of this technology should be considered, however.

An aberration of a given gene in an individual does not necessitate that the associated genetic disease will always be present. This phenomenon has been described as the "incomplete penetrance" of the disease. Two individuals may inherit the same genetic defect and yet one may develop the associated disease syndrome while the other does not. In addition, the severity of the associated disease syndrome may vary greatly among different afflicted individuals. Environmental and other, as yet, undefined factors often are important contributors in the disease process. These phenomena are significant in the potential for over-reliance on genetic testing to diagnose a disease state. A test may be "positive" in an individual who is not afflicted with a disease.

The utilization of genetic testing for discriminatory employment or insurance purposes is an important consideration as erroneous conclusions drawn from such studies could have damaging implications for individuals.[19] The privacy of this information should be considered as the potential for discrimination, particularly in terms of insurance risk, will grow. As the number of available diagnostic tests increases, a growing segment of the population may find themselves assigned to high-risk health insurance groups, or deemed "uninsurable."

A social stigma is often attached to genetic disorders. The potential for isolation, humiliation, and generation of self-fulfilling prophecies based on a presumed "diagnostic" study has been well established (CEJA, 1991). The need for protection of individual privacy of such information is evident. Instances of forced disclosure of such information to others, against the patient's will, would be appropriate only under limited circumstances, such as those outlined by Annas and Elias (1990) in which: "1) there is high probability of harm, 2) harm to identifiable individuals is serious, and 3) precautions are taken to limit disclosure to appropriate genetic information."

Genetic technology has enhanced our ability to diagnose disorders at an increasingly early stage. The ability to recognize the limitations of such testing is important. Over-reliance on genetic test results and indiscriminate dissemination of such information could be misused to deem an individual "unfit" or "uninsurable," rather than guiding appropriate medical care. The Working Group on Human Genome Mapping (CIOMS, 1991) concluded: "(a)n adequately prepared scientific, medical and lay community is the best defense against misuse of the information and the best assurance that the information and technology will be used in a way that preserves the dignity of the individual."

Conclusions

Gene therapy may provide an important new modality for the treatment of human diseases. In addition to the treatment of congenital deficiencies of a necessary protein, human gene therapy may provide pharmacologic production of a wide range of therapeutic proteins within the body. The ethical foundation upon which human gene therapy is built is the relief of human suffering. The future importance of this field in the medical armamentarium will depend on the development of the available technology and societal choices. Continued research will be necessary to allow for progress in overcoming the logistic obstacles presently hindering more wide-reaching applications. Accumulation of experience will allow for a more thorough assessment of the risks associated with gene therapy and enhance the ability to identify suitable target diseases. Regulatory oversight needs to be flexible in this developing field and sensitive to the impact of excessive restrictions. Public discussion of the broad implications of these endeavors will help to allow appropriate advancement of the science.

Notes

1. See, for example, Eglitis, M. A., and Anderson, W. F. (1988), "Retroviral vectors for introduction of genes into mammalian cells," *Biotechniques*, 6(7): 608–14.

2. An overview of the debates and controversy leading to the first gene therapy as presented in Carmen (1992), Roberts (1989), and Roberts, L. (1989), *Science*, 243: 734.

3. The study protocol is reprinted in Brenner, M. K., et al. (1991), *Human Gene Therapy*, 2: 137–59.

4. The study protocol is reprinted in Santana, V. M., et al. (1991), *Human Gene Therapy*, 2: 257–72.

5. The study protocol is reprinted in Deisseroth, A. B., et al. (1991), *Human Gene Therapy*, 2: 359–76.

6. The study protocol is reprinted in Cornetta, K., et al. (1992), *Human Gene Therapy*, 2: 305–18.

7. The study protocol is reprinted in Ledley, F. D., et al. (1991), *Human Gene Therapy*, 2: 331–58.

8. The study protocol is reprinted in Wilson, J. M., et al. (1992), *Human Gene Therapy*, 3: 179–222.

9. The study protocol is reprinted in Hsueh, J. L., et al. (1992), *Human Gene Therapy*, 3: 543–52.

10. The study protocol is reprinted in Nabel, G. J., et al. (1992), *Human Gene Therapy*, 3: 399–410.

11. Preclinical experiments are reported in: Culver, K. W., Ram, Z., Wallbridge, S., Ishi, H., Oldfield, E. H., and Blaese, R. M. (1992), "In vivo gene transfer with retroviral vector-producing cells for treatment of experimental brain tumors," *Science*, 256: 1550–52 and Short, M. P., Choi, B.C., Lee, J. K., Malick, A., Breakefield, X. O., and Martuz, R. L. (1990), "Gene delivery to glioma cells in rat brain by grafting of a retrovirus packaging cell line," Journal of Neuroscience Research, 27(3): 427–39.

12. The study protocol is reprinted in Riddell, S. R., et al. (1992), *Human Gene Therapy*, 3: 319–38.

13. For review articles on the potential applications of gene therapy, see: Friedman, T. (1989), "Progress toward human gene therapy," *Science*, 244: 1275–81; Kohn, D. B. and Kantoff, P. F. (1989), "Potential applications of gene therapy," *Transfusion*, 29(9): 812–20; Kohn, D. B., Anderson, W. F., and Blaese, R. M. (1989), "Gene therapy for genetic diseases," *Cancer Investigations*, 7(2): 179–92; and Anderson, W. F. (1984), "Prospects for human gene therapy," *Science*, 226: 401–409.

14. For a review of this topic see Weinberg, R. A. (1991), "Tumor suppressor genes," *Science*, 254: 1138–46.

15. See Department of Health and Human Services, Regulations for Protection of Human Subjects, 45 Code of Fed. Reg., Part 46.

16. Center for Biologics Evaluation and Research, Food and Drug Administration. "Draft Points to consider in human somatic cell therapy and gene therapy." Division of Biological Investigational New Drugs, Room 1-29, HFB-230, 12420 Parklawn Drive, Rockville, MD, 20852. Reprinted in *Human Gene Therapy*, 2: 251–56, 1991.

17. Recombinant DNA Advisory Committee, National Institutes of Health. "Points to consider in the design and submission of human somatic cell

gene therapy protocols." Fed. Reg. 54, no. 169, pp. 36698–703, September 1, 1989. Reprinted in *Human Gene Therapy*, 1: 93–103, 1990.

18. An overview of the aftermath of a recombinant bacterial genetic proposal is presented in Mackler (1990).

19. See CEJA, (1991) and accompanying editorial by Juengst, E. T. (1991), "Priorities in professional ethics and social policy for human genetics," *JAMA* 266(13): 1835–36.

References

Anderson, W. F. (1992). Human gene therapy. *Science*, 256: 808–13.

Annas, G. J., and Elias, S. (1990). Legal and ethical implications of fetal diagnosis and gene therapy. *American Journal of Medical Genetics*, 35: 215–18.

Areen, J., and King, P. (1990). Legal regulation of human gene therapy. *Human Gene Therapy*, 1: 151–61.

Bandara, G., Robbins, P. D., Georgescu, H. I., Mueller, G. M., Glorioso, J. C., and Evans, C. H. (1992). Gene transfer to synoviocytes: Prospects for gene treatment or arthritis. *DNA Cell Biol.*, 11(3): 227–31.

Bank, A., Markowitz, D., and Lerner, N. (1989). Gene transfer: a potential approach to gene therapy for sickle cell disease. Annals of the New York Academy of Sciences, 37–43.

Capecchi, M. R. (1989). Altering the genome by homologous recombination. *Science*, 244: 1288–92.

Carmen, I. H. (1992). Debates, divisions, and decisions: Recombinant DNA Advisory Committee (RAC) authorization of the first human gene transfer experiments. *American Journal of Human Genetics*, 50: 245–60.

Carter, C. O. (1977). Monogenetic disorders. *Journal of Medical Genetics*, 14: 316–20.

CEJA (Council on Ethical and Judicial Affairs, American Medical Association) (1991). Use of genetic testing by employers. *JAMA*, 266(13): 1827–30.

Childs, B. (1988). Molecular genetics in medicine. Introduction. Progress in Medical Genetics. 7:1–16.

CIOMS (Council for International Organizations of Medical Sciences) (1991). Genetic ethics and human values: Human genome mapping. Bankowski, Z., and Capron, A. M., eds. Geneva. *Human Gene Therapy*, 2: 123–29.

Deaths following elixir of sulfanilamide—Massengill (editorial) (1937). *JAMA*, 109: 1367.

Dichek, D. A., Neville, R. F., Zweibel, J. A., Freeman, S. M., Leon, M. B., and Anderson, W. F. (1989). Seeding of intravascular stents with genetically engineered endothelial cells. *Circulation*, 80(5): 1347–53.

Epstein, S. L. (1991). Regulatory concerns in human gene therapy. *Human Gene Therapy*, 2: 243–49.

Faraji-Shadan, F., Stubbs, J. D., and Bowman, P. D. (1990). A putative approach for gene therapy against human immunodeficiency virus (HIV). *Medical Hypotheses*, 32(2): 81–84.

Freese, A. and Geller, A. (1991). Infection of cultures striatal neurons with a defective HSV-1 vector: Implications for gene therapy. Nucleic Acids Research, 19(25): 7219–23.

Gage, F. H., Rosenberg, M. B., Tuszynski, M. H., Yoshida, K., Armstrong, D. M., Hayes, R. C., and Friedmann, T. (1990). Gene therapy in the CNS: Intracerebral grafting of genetically modified cells. Progress in Brain Research 86: 205–217.

Geller, A. I., Keyomarsi, K., Bryan, J., and Pardee, A. B. (1990). An efficient deletion mutant packaging system for defective herpes simples virus vectors: Potential applications to human gene therapy and neuronal physiology. *Proceedings of the National Academy of Science*, 87(22): 8950–54.

Gelling, E. M. K., and Cannon, P. R. (1938). Pathologic effects of elixir of sulfanilamide (diethylene glycol) poisoning. *JAMA*, 111: 919.

Golde, D. W. (1991). The stem cell. *Scientific American*, December 1991: 86–93.

Green, E. D., and Waterston, R. H. (1991). The human genome project: Prospects and implications for clinical medicine. *JAMA*, 266(14): 1966–75.

Jolly, D. J. (1991). HIV infection and gene transfer technology. *Human Gene Therapy*, 2: 111–12.

Kahn, P. (1992). Germany's gene law begins to bite. *Science*, 255: 524–94.

Kantoff, P. W., Freeman, S. M., and Anderson, W. F. (1988). Prospects for gene therapy for immunodeficiency diseases. Annual Review of Immunology, 6: 581–94.

Lung, H. Y., Cornelius, J. G., and Peck, A. B. (1991). Cloning and expression of the oxalyl-CoA decarboxylase gene from the bacterium, Oxalobacter formigenes: Prospects for gene therapy to control Ca-oxalate kidney stone formation. *American Journal of Kidney Disease*, 17(4): 381–85.

Mackler, B. F. (1990). Relationship between public concerns and regulation oversight of human gene transfer therapy. *Human Gene Therapy*, 1: 191–92.

Morgan, R. A., Looney, D. J., Muenchau, D. D., Wong-Staal, F., Gallo, R. C., and Anderson, W. F. (1990). Retroviral vectors expressing soluble CD4: A potential gene therapy for AIDS. AIDS Research and Human Retroviruses, 6(2): 183–91.

Nadkarni, K. S., Datar, R. H., and Rao, S. G. (1991). Antisense RNA therapy for CML—an hypothesis. *Medical Hypotheses*, 35(4): 307–10.

Palmer, J. G. (1991). Liability considerations presented by human gene therapy. *Human Gene Therapy*, 2: 235–42.

Ramsey, P. *The Patient As a Person* (New Haven: Yale University Press, 1970). 239–75.

Roberts, L. (1989). Ethical questions haunt new genetic technologies. *Science*, 243: 1134–36.

Rosenberg, S. A., Aebersold, P., Cornetta, K., Kasid, A., Morgan, R. A., Moen, R., Karson, E. M., Lotze, M. T., Yang, J. C., Topalian, S. L., Merino, M. J., Culver, K., Miller, A.D., Blaese, R. M., and Anderson, W. F. (1990). Gene transfer into humans—immunotherapy of patients with advanced melanoma using tumor-infiltrating lymphocytes modified by retroviral gene transduction. *New England Journal of Medicine*, 323(9): 570–78.

Rosenfeld, M. A., Yoshimura, K., Trapnell, B.C., Yoneyama, K., Rosenthal, E. R., Dalemans, W., Fukayama, M., Bargon, J., Stier, L. E., Stratford-Perricaudet, L., Perricaudert, M., Guggino, W. B., Pavirani, A., Lecocq, J-P., and Crystal, R. G. (1992). In vivo transfer of the human cystic fibrosis transmembrane conductance regulator gene to the airway epithelium. *Cell*, 658: 143–55.

Sun, M. (1981). Cline loses two NIH grants. *Science*, 214: 1220.

Tremisis, P. J., and Bich-Thuy, L. (1991). Restoration of high immunoglobulin gene expression in chronic lymphoid leukemia: A possible application for gene therapy. *Cell Immunology*, 135(2): 326–34.

Walters, L. (1986). The ethics of human gene therapy. *Nature*, 32: 225–27.

Four

The Genome Project and Health Services for Minority Populations

Herbert Nickens

Human genetics, as one of the "sciences of inequality," entwines society's racial/ethnic and economic biases with any genetic differences that can be detected, particularly if any of these differences are differentially distributed by race, ethnicity, or class. Numerous historical examples show what happens when genetics are drawn into arguments over the causes of social inequalities. The Human Genome Project (HGP) has the potential to specify at an unprecedented level of detail the differences among human beings. This information will be introduced into a United States social context which: (1) already has a long and disturbing history of drawing sharp distinctions among our citizens on the basis of race and ethnicity, and (2) has a long tradition of belief in biological determinism. Scientific theories and data have often been used to buttress prevailing biases. Some have asked whether the HGP may create a new "biologic underclass." This chapter will identify possible "danger zones" in which information from the Genome Project could be used in invidious ways with regard to racial/ethnic minorities.

Assuring that scientific information is not abused requires examining the seemingly unthinkable, or at least unlikely. Reading this chapter requires from the reader a willing suspension of disbelief. We must project former and current racial problems in the United States into a future of dramatically increased capability to specify the genetic make-up of individuals. We must imagine a future in which a blood, tissue, or amniotic fluid sample is all that is required to probe for a wide variety of genetic traits, including those that cause or predispose individuals to diseases, conditions, or merely traits. Many of these genes are likely to appear in different proportions in different racial or ethnic groups. This creates a world where, even *in utero*, important parts of an individual's future can be glimpsed.

A second challenge in constructing this chapter is that the heterogeneity concealed within this unitary term—minority—makes this discussion very unwieldy. While there is a core of "minority-ness" that can be characterized, the historical and social realities for minority groups and sub-groups are extremely varied. This chapter does not provide sufficient room to explore how the various minority sub-groups may interact with the information from the Human Genome Project to produce different outcomes. Because many of the prominent historical examples of presumed genetic inferiority have involved African Americans, I will more often use these to illustrate potential problems. Where possible scenarios seem more likely to involve other minority groups, those will be explored. No claim is made, however, to cover the point of view of all minority groups.

A final challenge in reading this chapter is to appreciate the vulnerability that is an intrinsic part of minority-ness. There are two parts to this vulnerability. One is the sense on the part of minorities that the majority world is hostile and dangerous to them and to their interests. The second part is to appreciate that historically there have been many, many instances which confirmed that minorities in the United States do occupy a perilous status. While the latter point should need no examples, the first point may. In a *Newsweek* poll a small but significant proportion of black adults (7 to 16 percent) blamed a racist conspiracy for drug abuse, AIDS, high crime rates, broken families, teen pregnancy, poor education, unemployment, and lack of black-owned business.[1] This is the volatile milieu into which the HGP will be introduced. Viewed in this context, majority scientists' exuberant proclamations that the HGP will produce the "Rosetta stone"[2] of life sound naive and insensitive.

Current Demographics

Any discussion of minority Americans must include some indication of how problematic the concept of "minorities" is. First of all, the term "minorities" only makes sense as a construct in relationship to a "majority." Grouping together the United States' minority populations bundles groups of extraordinary diversity. Second, any characterization of racial/ethnic minorities in the United States must acknowledge change in response to demographic, political, economic, and social shifts. The prevailing paradigm for U.S. minority groups derives from African Americans because of their large population; the complexity and economic importance of the slave system and its culmination in the Civil War; the power of the legacy of slavery and the codification of Jim Crow status in *de jure* segregation laws; and the Civil Rights movement as a defining period in American history.

The federal government recognizes four minority groups in the United States: American Indians / Alaska Natives, Asian/Pacific Islanders, blacks, and Hispanics.[3] The way in which these four groups came to be so designated by the federal government is relevant to this chapter, but the story would take us too far from our central task. These four groups differ enormously from one another, and there is great diversity within each group.

In my view, we designate people as a racial/ethnic minority in the American context when they: (1) are a small proportion of the overall population; (2) have a history of past discrimination in the United States; (3) are persistently socioeconomically disadvantaged; and (4) are people of color, that is, not European, not Caucasian. Despite the history of discrimination and oppression against those of European origins such as Irish-Americans, a particular intensity persists about the valence attached to "colored" minorities. As we shall see, Asian/Pacific Islanders have higher family income and high school graduation rates[4] than whites, and at least in this regard no longer fit all of the above criteria for minority groups.

Asian/Pacific Islanders are currently the fastest-growing population in the United States, increasing 108 percent from 1980 to 1990 compared to an increase of 13 percent for blacks, 53 percent for Hispanics, 38 percent for American Indians, and 6 percent for whites. Immigration was a substantial contributor to the increases in both the Asian and Hispanic populations; a high fertility rate is an additional important contributor to population increases among Hispanics.

Asian/Pacific Islander populations are heterogeneous. They include well-established Asian-American populations which are more likely to be born in the United States, such as Japanese and to a lesser extent Chinese, Filipinos, and Asian Indians. The median family income for Asian/Pacific Islanders is higher than for other minority groups and whites, although this figure reflects a larger number of workers per household, which inflates family income data. Vietnamese have an aver-

Race and Ethnicity in the U.S., 1990

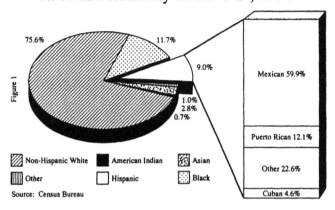

Figure 1

75.6%   11.7%

9.0%

1.0%
2.8%
0.7%

Mexican 59.9%

Puerto Rican 12.1%

Other 22.6%

Cuban 4.6%

Non-Hispanic White   American Indian   Asian

Other   Hispanic   Black

Source: Census Bureau

age family income which is about half that of the Asian/Pacific Islander population as a whole.[5]

Black Americans are currently the largest minority group in the United States. Diversity within black Americans is less overt than in other minority groups because of the homogenizing effect of the long-standing black presence in America. However, those blacks with origins in the former British West Indies have retained a discrete identity. More recently, substantial numbers of Haitian immigrants have come to the United States, particularly to Florida and New York. We do not have accurate data on the proportion of black Americans who are of West Indian or Haitian origins.

Approximately one-third of blacks live below the poverty level, and black unemployment has been approximately twice that of whites since 1940. In the past fifteen years the proportion of blacks who are poor has increased, while the black upper middle class has also increased substantially.

Hispanic Americans (see Figure 1) are the second-largest minority in the United States. As with Asian Americans, Hispanic Americans come from a variety of different countries. Three-fifths of Hispanic Americans are of Mexican origin. Hispanics are also diverse with regard to socioeconomic status, circumstances under which they came to the United States, and levels of acculturation. The "other Hispanic" component of this population is large and increasing very rapidly. This represents the increases in populations from Central and South America.

American Indians / Alaska Natives (AI/AN) are the smallest and perhaps most diverse of all American minority groups. About 2 million AI/AN are distributed among almost 500 tribes and village units. Of

Table 1: Selected Indicators of Well-Being for Minorities and Whites: Infant Mortality (IM), Poverty, and High School Graduation Rates

	IM ratio[7] (minor., white)	poverty rates (1988)[8]	high school grad. rates[9]
whites	1.00	10.1%	82.5%
blacks	1.05	31.6%	77.0%
Hispanics	Mex.Am .99 P.R 1.42	26.8%	54.5%
Asian P/I	.95	10.3%[10][a]	70%(f), 80%(m)[a]
AI/AN	1.53	23.7%[8][a]	56%[a]

[a] 1980 data

these, about half of the AI/AN population does not live on reservations. Overall AI/AN poverty rates are similar to those of Hispanics and blacks.

Even in this era when multiculturalism has become a buzzword, many people believe that minority groups have similar indices of well-being, perhaps with the exception of Asians, who carry the opposite burden—that of being seen as the "model minority." Table 1 contains selected indicators of well-being to offer further contrasts among minority groups and the majority. Infant mortality rates (IMRs) were chosen as the health indicator because they are widely accepted as a good measure of the overall well-being of a population. Moreover, the overall relative health status of these groups as measured by mortality rates parallels the pattern of the IMRs, with the exception of Asians, whose overall mortality rates are substantially lower than for any other group.[6] Ratios were used because our interest here is relative status rather than absolute numbers. What we see is a gradient of disadvantage, with blacks having the worst IMRs, then AI/AN, with Asians, whites and Mexican Americans having similar rates.

Poverty is generally measured by some combination of income, educational attainment, and occupation, all of which are highly intercorrelated. Many argue that poverty, not race/ethnicity, determines life chances for Americans. However, if we attempt to correlate the ranking of IMRs with the poverty rates in the next column and high school graduation rates in the far right column, it is very difficult to argue for a *simplistic* relationship between health status and poverty. Mexican Americans present the most striking incongruities: surprisingly good health status, high poverty rates, and very low educational attainment.

It is also important to note the contrast between Puerto Rican health status and that of Mexicans.

Lessons of History

When thinking about the egregious involvement of science in racist enterprises, examples from Nazi Germany easily come to mind. However, it is clear that in the United States race and science have intertwined to produce outrageous outcomes. I will offer three cases:

The Tuskegee Experiment

The Tuskegee Experiment began in the early 1930s under the auspices of the U.S. Public Health Service as an outgrowth of a syphilis control project in the rural South. It was originally intended to be a study of less than a year to investigate the natural history of syphilis in blacks and to investigate whether there are racial differences in the manifestations of the disease. The study lasted forty years, and its participants were observed untreated over that time period. What made the study so sinister was not only the withholding of informed consent and treatment from the participants, but the fact that black institutions were brought into the study to provide legitimacy and to maintain continued participation of the subjects. In fact, the same black public health nurse was kept as the primary contact person throughout the study. The study was terminated in 1972 after exposure in the news media. The Tuskegee experiment contributed directly to the current comprehensive federal regulations regarding the protection of human subjects in research. But the Tuskegee experiment also left a legacy in the black community of bitter mistrust of science and experimentation.[11]

Genetic Theories of Intelligence

The interest in measuring intelligence has been intense in the United States since early in this century, when the first intelligence tests were developed. Measurements of intelligence were quickly drawn into social conflicts when intelligence scores of recent European immigrant groups were compared to those of white Americans who had immigrated earlier. This activity was greatly facilitated by the massive intelligence testing by the U.S. Army among soldiers in World War I. Recent European immigrants scored lower than immigrants who had been in the

United States for a longer period of time. While blacks as a whole scored low on these tests, even lower than those of Italian, Polish, or Russian national origin, the scores of northern blacks were higher than these recent immigrants. Interestingly, Sowell has shown that the IQs of groups have tended to shift over time, with those of recent immigrants rising toward the national average.[12]

The belief that different races are endowed with different levels of a quality called intelligence has persisted. In the late 1960s and early 1970s Arthur Jensen and William Shockley brought the battle about race and IQ boiling to the surface. At a time when the Great Society programs of President Johnson sought to achieve racial equality, Jensen stated, "we are left with various lines of evidence . . . (which) make it a not unreasonable hypothesis that genetic factors are strongly implicated in the average Negro-white intelligence difference."[13] William Shockley, whose fame resulted from his invention of the transistor, had long asserted the genetic inferiority of blacks. He seized on Jensen's article and added more fuel to the fire, suggesting that sterilization of those with low intelligence might avoid, " . . . retrogressive evolution through disproportionate reproduction of genetically disadvantaged."[14]

Jensen, Shockley, and their defenders were prevented from speaking on many college campuses and other forums because of protests, or were shouted down when they did appear. The Jensen-Shockley episode exposed the wellspring of belief that social inequalities among races must flow from innate (genetic) inferiority. At the same time it made clear how volatile public discussion of innate differences can be.

Sickle Cell Anemia

In the 1940s hemoglobin was the first molecule in which an association was made between a mutant gene and a specific amino acid substitution. Sickle cell anemia (SC) became overtly political in the 1970s. Four black Army recruits died suddenly during basic training at Fort Bliss, Texas. The recruits were heterozygous for SC and Fort Bliss is 4,060 feet above sea level. The cases were described first in the *New England Journal of Medicine* and then picked up by the national press.[15] An accompanying editorial in the *New England Journal* called sickle cell the most neglected major health problem in the United States. One of the authors stated that since the deaths he had screened all black recruits for SC.[16]

The SC controversy from the beginning contained conflicting messages, which are generalizable to genetic diseases in minorities. On the one hand there was outrage about the neglect of this disease and great agitation for research and widespread testing for SC. On the other hand the proposals to screen couples for SC before marriage, the exclusion of SC carriers from certain occupations, and the possibility of increased insurance rates raised questions of racial discrimination.

With SC, examples of these conflicting messages are abundant. In the early 1970s federal legislation was passed to support the creation of research and testing programs for SC. Fundraisers were held by celebrities to support SC programs. The governing board of the New York Health and Hospitals Corporation called for testing of all black children admitted to one of the HHC hospitals,[17] although later this effort was judged not feasible.[18] At the same time, an 18-member group concerned with bioethics raised caution about mass screening for genetic diseases like SC, including the importance of screening being voluntary, explaining the meaning of a positive result, and confidentiality.[19] Passionate advocacy for SC programs existed side-by-side with denunciations of genetic counseling as a "white plot" to carry out genocide against blacks.[20]

SC has at least two lessons for us: (1) genetic disease can serve both as a rallying point for drawing attention to the needs of a group, and at the same time a source of increased stigmatization with imputation of innate defectiveness; and (2) during periods where knowledge about such a disease is incomplete—how at-risk are carriers of SC?—there is great opportunity for serious policy errors. The HGP will create myriad opportunities to prove the adage, "a little knowledge is a dangerous thing."

A Proposed Conceptual Framework for Understanding the Relationship between Stigma, Minorities, and Genetic Information

The mixture of science and race can produce results which are irrational and abusive, and which nonetheless, have the legitimacy conferred by science. Minority status carries with it a certain stigma, hence a landmark book on the psychology of race was named *The Mark of Oppression*.[21] As with many other aspects of race/ethnicity, such stigma is never far from consciousness for minorities and is one of the lenses through which life is perceived. Not surprisingly, awareness of this stigma is for white Americans much less a part of everyday experience, but certainly informs attitudes toward racial/ethnic minorities. This visceral reaction made the "Willie Horton" ads used by the Bush campaign in the 1988 elections devastatingly effective. This same effect can be seen in public discussions about welfare or out-of-wedlock child bearing.

Increasingly we are seeing stigma played out with regard to health. The major chronic diseases—for example, cardiovascular disease, cancer and diabetes—are now the most important killers of Americans, including minority Americans. The challenges of these chronic diseases are sometimes dubbed the second public health revolution, to contrast it with the "first revolution," the dramatic reduction in deaths from infectious diseases which occurred in the hundred years following the Civil War. Lifestyle and behavior are central to the acquisition and development of major chronic diseases. Superimposed on this are two other current public health problems: the explosive increases in HIV infection, which disproportionately afflicts already stigmatized groups—homosexual men and minorities; and the increasing rates and flamboyance of minority homicides. Behavioral choices are also the proximate cause of high HIV infection and homicide rates.

HIV and homicide raise yet another complexity in our consideration of stigma: some behaviors do violate our collective sense of morality. Homicide is wrong. Knowingly exposing another person to HIV is wrong. Thus, in judging these questions of stigma and discrimination we must look to see whether these moral standards may be applied more harshly or inflexibly, such that the same behavior is judged differently when minorities are involved.

My hypothesis is that with regard to minority populations and genetic disease there is a convergence of at least four themes which together create a powerful potential for discrimination and stigma:

(1) Because of the stigma associated with minority status, any disvalued trait associated with minorities has that negative valence amplified. The HGP will offer numerous opportunities for further stigmatization of minorities.

(2) There is a substantial lack of identification with minorities on the part of the majority; diseases or problems of minorities are seen as afflicting "them" not "us."

(3) Our society puts tremendous value on personal responsibility for and control over our behavior, and health promotion / disease prevention activities intensify this tendency. Diseases which are the result of behavior are viewed very negatively.

(4) Eugenics, social Darwinism,[22] and "racial hygiene"[23] have historically been strong movements in the United States.

For most genes, and clusters of genes, minorities will be found to have the same distribution of base sequences and phenotypic variations as for whites. For some genes, and clusters of genes, minorities will be found to have a different distribution of variation. There is potential for discrimination and stigma in both circumstances. There is potential for differential treatment for minorities with "defective genes," even for those traits for which minorities have a similar distribution of variation as that for majority populations; and certainly there is potential for stigma for those negative traits or diseases which are strongly associated with minorities. As a way to begin to look at the potential for discrimination and stigma we will examine two current examples, (a) a comparison of cystic fibrosis (CF) and sickle cell, and (b) low birthweight (LBW).

CF is the most common genetic disease among whites. Carriers of the CF gene are virtually all white. SC is the most common genetic disease among blacks. The frequency of homozygous CF children among whites is lower than the frequency of homozygous SC children among blacks—1/1600–2000 births versus 15/1000.[24, 25] Moreover, there are 50% more individuals with SC disease in the United States than those with CF.[26] Both diseases manifest themselves early in life and kill many of those afflicted before they reach middle age. It is therefore interesting to look at two important differences in these diseases: the attitudes toward those with these diseases and the relative public and private funding for research.

It is difficult to ascertain public attitudes toward those with CF or SC, in part because most Americans know little about them. This author does have substantial anecdotal experience regarding the attitudes of majority health care workers toward the two groups. In general, persons with CF are regarded with compassion, consistent with how one would expect health care workers to view those with a genetic, chronic, and fatal disease. Persons with SC disease are regarded somewhat more negatively, and those negative sentiments tend to be organized around the intermittent severe pain associated with SC disease. Health care workers often question whether those with SC disease are having "real" pain or exhibiting analgesic drug-seeking behavior. We do not know whether these negative attitudes are independent of the fact that those with SC disease are virtually all black, while those with CF are virtually all white.

The relative funding levels of CF and SC are not ambiguous. SC research was allocated almost $18 million by the NIH in Fiscal Year 1992 House of Representatives Appropriations Committee.[27] For the same year, CF research at the NIH was budgeted for $46 million.[28] In addition, the Cystic Fibrosis Foundation in 1990 provided $18 million in research support.[29]

Low birthweight provides a slightly different insight into the interaction between race and genetic disease. Low birthweight is the most important contributor to infant mortality. For as long as we have had national data, black infant mortality has been much higher than that for whites. In the past forty years infant mortality rates (IMRs) for whites and blacks have decreased but slightly more rapidly for whites, such that blacks now have IMRs more than twice that for whites. Low birthweight has not significantly decreased in the past twenty years, and improvements in IMRs have been achieved largely by high technology interventions that improve the survival of small infants. The issue of high IMRs among blacks is a source of outrage for critics of our current health and social policies and embarrassment for the defenders of those policies. It has often been suggested that at least part of the higher LBW rates among blacks may be genetic, and this possibility was raised again in a 1986 study.[30]

Such a finding can encourage abdication of social responsibility by reasoning that if a condition is genetic, then we are helpless and blameless. Countering this view Dr. Wendy Baldwin wrote an a companion editorial, " . . . great strides can be made in applying what we already know how to do (to reduce low birthweight). Will this ensure the end of disparities between groups? No . . . We have much to learn, but much to do while we are learning."[31]

The stigmatizing nature of genetic traits is not an all-or-none phenomenon. Table 2 lays out possible variations in the potential of different kinds of genetically coded traits to elicit negative labeling. Please note that in creating this chart, no effort was made to limit examples to those traits which have already been proven to be under some genetic influence.

Potential for Discrimination

One of the cross-cutting problems that will arise in all of these areas is our limited knowledge. Once we have the capacity to document genetic differences among individuals, and among groups, there is an almost irresistible tendency to make something of those differences. This occurred in workplace testing for glucose-6-phosphate dehydrogenase deficiency (G6PD) and SC in the 1970s.[32,33] Once we have documented the genetic differences among populations, it may take an extraordinary amount of research to find out with any precision what those differences mean. The disease-related genes which have now been located were largely found because investigators were working backward from a disease expressed in a phenotype to a location of a gene, and in some cases determining the disease gene's DNA sequence. For most diseases that

Table 2:
Potential of Different Types of Genes for Stigma/Discrimination

Type of Trait for which Gene Codes	Example	Potential for Stigma/ Discrimination
physical appearance	skin color	high
not visible, no substantive implications	ability to taste a given chemical	low
addiction	alcoholism	high
response to medication	differing response to antihypertensive agents	low
physical/mental capabilities	hand-eye coordination	variable
susceptibility to environmental exposures	development of disease with exposure to chemicals in the workplace	high
behavior	impulse control	high
disease	sickle cell anemia	variable

have a genetic basis, that genetic basis is a polygenetic one, such as in-sulin-dependent diabetes mellitus or coronary heart disease, and will present even more of a challenge to scientists. The HGP data will present scientists with a vast amount of raw data about genetic locations and DNA sequences for which the clinical significance will be unknown. This is particularly true since an estimated 90–95 percent of the human genome is estimated to be "junk" DNA, which appears to not code for proteins and whose function is unknown. This suggests a period of perhaps decades during which our knowledge of genetic mapping and sequencing may be complete, but our knowledge of the significance of that information will be incomplete. If history is any guide, this time of incomplete information will function like a Rorschach—its meaning will be in the eye of the beholding society. For minorities this will be a perilous time.

Because there will be such a long period during which we will know the location and, later, sequences of genes, but our knowledge will be otherwise incomplete, it is important to review how genes behave in a real world population. Eight considerations have a direct influence:

1. Prevalence—how common are the various versions of the gene? If a particular version of the gene is problematic (e.g., causes a disease), how prevalent is it?
2. Racial/ethnic variation—is the gene distributed very differently

among different racial/ethnic groups; for example, common in one or more minorities, but rare among whites?

3. Effect of gene—is the gene associated with a disease, a condition, a differential response to medications or chemicals in the environment, or differential physical or mental capabilities? (See also Table 1.)

4. Variability in the expression of the gene—does the gene have complete penetrance or is the phenotypic expression highly variable? Does this variability not only include the intensity of the expression of the gene, but the age at which manifestations are likely to appear?

5. Absolute probability of those with the gene acquiring the disease—the absolute probability is the relative risk of acquiring the disease in the presence of the gene, combined with the prevalence of the disease in the population. Even with a high relative risk, a very rare disease may even be rare in those with the gene.

6. Modifiability of developing disease or condition—in the presence of the gene, can the disease or condition be modified, or even prevented?

7. Stigmatizing nature of disease or condition—does the disease have a minimal potential for stigma or is it potentially highly stigmatizing, such as a gene for alcoholism? (See also Table 1.)

8. Quality of evidence supporting the above—have the molecular biology, epidemiology, and clinical studies been done which confirm the type of questions asked above, or are the answers highly speculative?

In the balance of this chapter, I shall explore possible arenas of discrimination based on genetic information. The arenas that will be discussed are access to health care, and four other arenas with implications for access to health care, as well as broader implications for quality of life: the workplace, insurance, the welfare system, and the criminal justice system.

Access to Health Care

About one-third of Hispanics and one-quarter of blacks lack health insurance, compared to about one-eighth of whites (data on other minorities are not available). More striking is that even within economic groupings—the poor, near poor, and nonpoor—Hispanics and blacks are still more likely to be uninsured as compared to whites.[34]

Moreover, health insurance only provides the minimal "ticket" to obtain health care. Minorities with insurance are more likely to be insured through the Medicaid program, which provides severely limited access to care. Moreover, there is an increasingly robust literature showing that blacks, at least, have less access to a wide variety of therapies even when potential confounding variables such as type of insurance, whether one is insured at all, age, and social class are held constant.[35,36,37,38,39,40,41,42] This "therapeutic discrimination" probably arises from some combination of provider biases, subtle differences in sources of care, patient behavior, and regional variations. Unfortunately, there is every reason to expect that as new gene-based therapies become available, blacks, and perhaps other minorities, will have less access to these therapies as they now do to the numerous therapies referenced above.

All of these current limitations on access to care for minorities will operate with respect to gene-related services. However, not only will one's ability to access health care affect access to genetic services, genetic information has the potential to influence access to care both through denial of insurance coverage and more subtle shunting and avoidance of patients with genetic predispositions to certain conditions. This shunting and avoidance could operate through economic incentives (health care for these persons could prove expensive) or because of personal revulsion at treating patients with certain diseases.

At the time of the preparation of this manuscript our nation is once again considering whether health insurance should be provided to all citizens. It is my opinion that—as at other times during this century when this question was being debated—the outcome of this health care reform effort will fall considerably short of universal coverage. To the degree that health care reform fails to produce health insurance that is invulnerable to job or income changes, minorities' access to care will continue to be particularly fragile. However, even for minorities who have health insurance, access to genetic counseling may prove a mixed blessing. There are at least three components to this: (1) these insured minorities may have less access to genetic counseling as they now have to other services as discussed above; (2) there may be bias on the part of the counseling system which may subtly adjust the advice given to prospective mothers and fathers. Particularly in gray areas of knowledge, how the counselor views the client may change the recommendations and evaluation of risk. For example, about two-thirds of black children are born out of wedlock versus about one out of five for whites. While family context is a legitimate consideration, "illegitimacy" is a fertile area for prejudice; and (3) genetic counselors are likely to be unprepared for the variations of values by race/ethnicity or social class. A non-genetic example is many people's surprise at the willingness of minority HIV-positive mothers to carry a pregnancy to term despite a probability of about one in four of bearing an HIV-positive child. This decision can hinge on differences in perspective, including a different calculus regarding: risk and hazard, the burdens of a "defective" child, one's time horizon, and religious considerations.

Workplace

Workplace testing illustrates the dangers of the capacity to screen for genes without complete knowledge of the significance of those genes. Moreover, most health insurance is connected to employment. There are as yet no genes for which there is scientific consensus regarding the appropriateness of workplace testing.[43] It is also not clear what the current level of genetic testing is in the workplace. The Dupont company received a large amount of negative publicity more than a decade ago with regard to its testing of black employees for SC. Part of that negative publicity is illustrative of the discriminatory potential in workplace testing. SC is present in both black and white Mediterranean populations. Moreover, thalassemia and G6PD deficiency also occur in both populations and all three conditions theoretically could cause anemia in the presence of workplace chemicals. Even at the biggest Dupont plant in Deepwater, NJ, which had a substantial number of employees with Italian surnames, blacks were the only group singled out for genetic screening.[44]

In view of the generally negative fallout associated with the SC and G6PD testing efforts of the past, accurate current data on workplace testing are difficult to obtain. A 1982 Office of Technology Assessment survey of over 500 companies yielded 366 responses, of which only 6 companies acknowledged current testing, 17 stated they had done so in the past twelve years, and 55 said they would possibly test in the next five years.[45]

Minorities are at special risk with regard to workplace screening for several reasons:

1. Minorities disproportionately occupy lower skilled positions. This means that employers can readily find workers for positions; and that these jobs are more likely to involve exposure to chemicals, dust, and other workplace hazards for which a genetic susceptibility might be a concern.
2. Because of lower educational levels, minorities may be less aware of their rights, submitting to discriminatory testing or, because of lack of sophistication, might not even be aware that they are being tested.

3. Many minorities who are recent immigrants have limited English facility, and yet because of wishing to not appear incompetent, may accede to an employer's request without understanding the implications.
4. Many minorities who are not citizens or permanent residents may feel unwilling to assert their rights for fear of denial of citizenship or even deportation from the U.S. This is particularly problematic for those who are in the country illegally.
5. Racial/ethnic prejudices may lead employers to apply genetic testing procedures in a discriminatory way, much the same way that the likelihood of being tested for HIV in an emergency room is certainly highly dependent on whether the patient "looks like" one of the high-risk groups.

Insurance Screening

The HGP raises concerns about health insurance, as well as life or disability insurance. The theory behind insurance involves the spreading of risk among a population, with the payments of those who are well subsidizing the care of those who fall ill, become disabled, or die. Insurance companies are becoming increasingly aggressive in screening individuals and populations for risk-rating purposes with regard to health insurance.[46] Insurance companies, in general, now reserve the right to deny insurance or charge higher premiums based on pre-existing conditions. The HGP offers the potential to identify with new precision those who are likely to become ill, perhaps decades in the future, severely truncating the unpredictability which underlies the concept of insurance. As with workplace screening, the potential of HGP to distort the fundamental nature and hence availability of insurance is a generic problem. However, for the same reasons as stated under workplace screening, minorities are especially vulnerable to differential exclusion.

AFDC and Other Public Assistance Programs

Because of higher poverty rates, minorities are disproportionately involved with, and dependent on, public programs, including health services provided through the public health system and Medicaid. Though these programs provide important services, the fact that they serve disadvantaged populations has important consequences as well. For example, syphilis and gonorrhea are reportable conditions; therefore, cases are required to be reported to the health department both for possible follow-up (e.g., contact tracing) and for statistical purposes. However, it is widely recognized that there is substantial underreporting of cases of sexually transmitted diseases (STDs) seen in private physicians' offices as compared with public clinics.[47] Among other consequences, this results in distortion of STD rates by race/ethnicity.

If genetic information became widely used in medical settings or as screens for employment, it is likely that information regarding the genetic vulnerabilities of minorities would be relatively over-reported. This would be true because: (1) unfavorable genetic information is more likely to be concealed by private physicians; and (2) breaches of confidentiality and abuse of the information are more likely for public clinic patients.

Criminal Justice System

It is difficult to overestimate the role of the police and the correctional system in minority communities. In a study done by the Sentencing Project, one in four black men between the ages of 20–29 is under the control of the criminal justice system: either incarcerated, on parole, or on probation. The absolute number was 609,690—40 percent larger than the number in higher education. The comparable rates for young Hispanic men were one in ten, and one in 16 for young white men.[48] Not only does such a high incarceration rate radically distort the social and economic structure, it means that for those populations with high incarceration rates, prison policies hold sway over their lives. Moreover, in President Clinton's health proposal, prisoners along with illegal aliens were not to be covered by health insurance.[49]
A scenario:

> The year is 1998. Scientists have located a gene which they believe is related to excessive violence and diminished impulse control (known as the V-DIC gene). Congress, spurred on by a president who was elected in part because of a "get tough on crime" program, passes a law requiring that all federal prisoners be required to provide a blood sample for DNA testing. This DNA testing not only includes a test for the V-DIC gene, but also requires that DNA "fingerprints" be taken and kept on file for all habitual offenders. State legislators, sensing the popularity of this measure, quickly pass similar measures applying to their state and local prison populations. Since such DNA "fingerprints" can be obtained from minute traces of blood, semen, saliva, skin, and hair follicles, this information becomes a powerful new weapon in en-

couraging prisoners to "plead out" charges when they are arrested.

Civil libertarians and civil rights leaders argue in vain that these laws are discriminatory—the national prison population in 1998 is 70 percent minority and climbing. First, they argue that the V-DIC gene screening is unfair: (a) because the evidence linking the V-DIC gene to crime is still far from conclusive; and (b) the gene has a much higher frequency in black and Puerto Rican populations. Since much of the V-DIC basic science was done with prison populations with high proportions of individuals who are black and Puerto Rican, this finding of higher frequency is circular reasoning. Second, they argue that DNA fingerprinting does have a small error rate, which is markedly increased under the real-world conditions of collection of specimens at a crime scene.

These same civil rights leaders are particularly alarmed about the increasing popularity of proposals to test minority adolescents for the V-DIC gene and, for those testing positive, to structure special middle school and high school criminal behavior prevention classes for these youths so identified. To anyone who will listen they ask, "Where will this end?"

Conclusion

In many respects the procedures that have been developed to protect human subjects in research, and the bioethical deliberations around science, are reassuring for their thoughtfulness and generally meticulous application. However, society's latent bigotries, from which the scientific community itself is not immune, are a constant danger to distort scientific priorities and scientific information.

There is also the problem of what happens to scientific information in the "real world." As science becomes more sophisticated, our questions shift from what *can* we do, to what *should* we do? We need to develop better mechanisms to bring the public and their representatives into these discussions. Moreover, as we come to understand nature better, very few things can *never* happen. It is a question of probabilities. We have seen a number of bad policies created around HIV, such as premarital screening and proposed testing of all health care workers. In part, these policies flow from prejudices associated with AIDS. But they also result because the public, including public policymakers, need to be educated to evaluate risk, including appreciating the magnitude of the risks that we take every day.

I have no hope that prejudices can be made to disappear. What we can accomplish is to create frameworks that make it very difficult for latent prejudice to transform itself into policies or programs.

Notes

1. *Newsweek*, April 6, 1992, 22.

2. Gilbert, W., "Genome sequencing: Creating a new biology for the twenty-first century," *Issues in Science and Technology* (Spring 1987), 26–35.

3. U.S. Bureau of the Census, Press Release CB91-216, 1991. Please note: Unless otherwise indicated all demographic information from this section is derived from this source.

4. U.S. Department of Commerce, Bureau of the Census, Current Population Reports, P-20-459. The Asian and Pacific Islander Population in the United States: March 1991 and 1990. Washington, DC: U.S. Government Printing Office, 1992.

5. Gardner, R. W., Robey, B., and Smith, P. C., "Asian Americans: Growth, change, and diversity," *Population Bulletin*, 40(4) (1985).

6. Nickens, H. W., "The health status of minority populations in the United States," *Western Journal of Medicine* (July 1991), 27–32.

7. Kleinman, J. C., "1990 Infant mortality among minority groups," CDC Surveillance Summaries, MMWR 39(ss-3): 31–40.

8. Current Population Reports, Series P-60, No. 166. U.S. Bureau of the Census.

9. Carter, D. J., Wilson, R., *Minorities in Higher Education: 1991*, table 1. American Council on Education, January 1992.

10. 1980 Census of Population, vol. 1, chapter C (PC80-1-C) and vol. 2, chapter 1E (PC80-2-1E), U.S. Bureau of the Census.

11. Thomas, S. B., Quinn, S. C., "The Tuskegee syphilis study, 1932 to 1972: Implications for HIV education AIDS risk education programs in the black community," *American Journal of Public Health*, 1991; 80: 1498–1505.

12. Sowell, T., "Race and IQ reconsidered," 203–38, in Sowell, ed., *Essays and Data on American Ethnic Groups* (Washington, DC: Urban Institute, 1978).

13. Jensen, A. R., "How much can we boost IQ and scholastic achievement?" 1–123, in *Environment, Heredity, and Intelligence* (Cambridge, MA: Harvard Educational Review, 1969).

14. *New York Times*, December 5, 1973, c2, 38.

15. Jones, S. R., Binder, R. A., Donowho, E. M., "Sudden death in sickle-cell trait," *New England Journal of Medicine* 282: 323–25, 1970.

16. *New York Times*, Feb. 16, 1970, c2, 75.

17. *New York Times*, July 27, 1971, c1, 29.

18. *New York Times*, October 28, 1971, c6, 54.

19. *New York Times*, May 25, 1972, c1, 9.

20. *New York Times*, December 29, 1972, c5, 12.

21. Kardiner, A., Ovesey, L. *The Mark of Oppression: Explorations in the Personality of the American Negro* (New York: World Publishing, 1951).

22. Degler, C. N. *In Search of Human Nature: The Decline and Revival of Darwinism in American Social Thought* (Oxford University Press; NY, Oxford, 1991).

23. Proctor, R. *Racial Hygiene: Medicine under the Nazis* (Harvard University Press; Cambridge, MA, London, 1988).

24. Colten, H. R. "Cystic Fibrosis," chap. 209 in Wilson, J. D., Braunwald, E., Isselbacher, K. J., Petersdorf, R. G., Martin, J. B., Fauci, A. S., and Root, R. K., *Harrison's Principles of Internal Medicine* (NY: McGraw Hill, 1991).

26. *Newsweek*, August 31, 1987, 60.

27. Committee on Appropriation Hearings, House of Representatives, Appropriations for 1992, April 11, 1991, 821.

28. Ibid., 647.

29. Cystic Fibrosis Foundation, 1990 Annual Report.

30. Shiono, P. H., Klebanoff, M. A., Graubard, B. I., Berendes, and Rhoads, G. G., "Birth weight among women of different ethnic groups," *JAMA*, 1986; 255: 48–52.

31. Baldwin, W., "Half empty, half full: What we know about low birth weight among blacks," *JAMA*, 1986; 255: 86–88.

32. Stokinger, H. E., Scheel, L. D., "Hypersusceptibility and genetic problems in occupational medicine: A consensus report," *Journal of Occupational Medicine*, 15:7 (July 1973): 564–73.

33. Murray, T. H., "Warning: Screening workers for genetic risk," Hastings Center Report, February, 1983: 5–8.

34. The Robert Wood Johnson Foundation, "Access to health care: key indicators for policy" prepared by the Center of Health Economics Research, Princeton, NJ, November, 1993.

35. Bashur, R. L., Homan, R. K., Smith, D. G., "Beyond uninsured: Problems in access to care," *Medical Care*, 1994; 32: 409–19.

36. Kogan, M. D., Kotelchuck, M., Alexander, G. R., Johnson, W. E., "Racial disparities in reported prenatal care advice from health care providers," *American Journal of Public Health*, 1994; 84: 82–88.

37. Goldberg, K. C., Hartz, A. J., Jacobsen, S. J., Krakauer, H., Rimm, A. A., "Racial and community factors influencing coronary artery bypass graft surgery rates for all 1986 Medicare patients," *JAMA*, 1992; 267: 1473–77.

38. Wenneker, M. B. and Epstein, A. M., "Racial inequalities in the use of

procedures for patients with ischemic heart disease in Massachusetts,"
JAMA, 1989; 261: 253–57.

39. Buckle, J. M., Horn, S. D., Oates, V. M., and Abbey, H., "Severity of illness and resource use differences among white and black hospitalized elderly," *Archives of Internal Medicine*, 1992; 152: 1596–1603.

40. Moore, R. D., Stanton, D., Gopalan, R. and Chaisson, R. E., "Racial differences in the use of drug therapy for HIV disease in an urban community," *New England Journal of Medicine*, 1994; 330: 763–68.

41. Diehr, P., Yergan, J., Chu, J., Feigl, P., Glaefke, G., Moe, R., Bergner, M.,
and Rodenbaugh, J., "Treatment modality and quality differences for black
and white breast-cancer patients treated in community hospitals," *Medical
Care*, 1989; 27: 942–58.

42. Todd, K. H., Samaroo, N., Hoffman, J. R., "Ethnicity as a risk factor for
inadequate emergency department analgesia," *JAMA*, 1993; 269: 1537–39.

43. Johnson Foundation, "Access to health care."

44. *New York Times*, February 3–6, 1980.

45. U.S. Congress, Office of Technology Assessment, Genetic Monitoring and
Screening in the Workplace, OTA-BA-455 (Washington, DC: U.S. Government Printing Office, October 1990), 202.

46. Light, D. W., "The practice and ethics of risk-related health insurance,"
JAMA, 1992; 267: 2503–08.

47. Aral, S. O., and Holmes, K. K., "Epidemiology of sexually transmitted
diseases," in Holmes, K. K., Mardh, P. A., Sparling, P. F., and Wiesner,
P. J., eds., *Sexually Transmitted Diseases* (New York: McGraw Hill, 1984),
126–41.

48. Mauer, M., "Young black men and the criminal justice system: A growing
national problem," Sentencing Project, Washington, DC, 1990.

49. The Health Security Act. The White House, 1993.

Five

Genetics and Reproductive Decision Making

Mary Anne Bobinski

The Human Genome Project (HGP) will have dramatic implications for reproductive decision making. In its initial stages, mapping the human genome primarily will increase our knowledge about the risks of reproducing. Genetic testing before attempted reproduction might be used to identify a large number of genetic conditions or predispositions that might be transferred to our offspring. After conception, the fetus' genetic code could be examined for genetic conditions, whether inherited or the result of mutation. Genetic testing will provide information that can be used in a broad range of decisions, ranging from whether to attempt to procreate to deciding whether to obtain an abortion once a pregnancy has occurred.

As the project progresses, knowledge about genetic risks will be accompanied by techniques designed to ameliorate or eliminate the negative consequences of genetic pathology. Genetic engineering could be used to alter the genetic characteristics of gametes or of fertilized ova, eliminating certain genetic conditions. Medical researchers may develop genetic therapies that counteract or diminish the negative effects of certain genetic variations. Somewhat more controversially, parents may be able to decide to "improve" the "normal" genotype by producing children who are taller, smarter, or more athletic (Purdy, 1995).

The expansion of knowledge and technology will produce three critical and interrelated questions. First, will the available genetic technologies provide useful information to men and women considering whether or not to reproduce? Second, will the decision whether or not to use genetic technology remain with the individual or will it be assumed by the government? Third, will the government attempt to regulate procreative choice once genetic information is known?

This chapter focuses on both the utility of genetic testing to potential reproducers and the ability to make procreative choices free from governmental interference. The first part describes the "value" of pre-conception and post-conception genetic testing from the standpoint of the individual choosing whether or not to undergo testing. The second part explores the ability of the state to require use of or to limit access to different types of genetic testing services. The third part of the chapter will focus on the ability of the state to regulate the "outcomes" of genetic technology by placing restrictions on individuals' procreative liberty. In the final part, I conclude that the HGP presents the possibility of greatly improving the procreative lives of men, women, and their children. Power is the most important issue in determining whether our hopes become reality. Positive reproductive health outcomes are most likely to come from giving potential parents—rather than governmental entities—the power to determine whether or not to make use of genetic technology and information.

The Value of Genetic Testing in Reproductive Decision Making

The Value of Pre-Conception Testing[1]

There are about 5,700 known genetic disorders (Connor and Ferguson-Smith, 1993), about 300 of which currently are detectable with genetic testing (Maddalena, Bick and Schulman, 1992). The HGP is rapidly expanding the list of genetic abnormalities known to be associated with particular disabling conditions. Pre-conception genetic testing is an important method of providing information to prospective reproducers about the likelihood that they will pass on some genetic characteristic to their offspring. Historically, information about an individual's genetic make-up could be obtained through an examination of the person's medical record and an analysis of his or her family genetic history. A family history of a particular disorder, for example, would mean that there was an elevated risk that the individual might be a carrier who could pass the condition to a new generation. This information is of limited value, however, in large part because it does not generally reveal

Table 1: Some Current Screening Tests (Harman, 1995)

Tested Group	Condition or Trait
African Americans	sickle cell
Ashkenazic Jews	Tay-Sachs
Mediterranean descent	β-Thalessemia
Southeast Asians	α-Thalessemia
Family history of CF; or, possibly, whites of northern European ancestry	cystic fibrosis

that the interested subject is in fact a carrier of a particular trait. For some conditions, carrier status can be revealed by an individual's own biochemical attributes.

More recently, geneticists have developed a number of different tests for potentially disabling genetic conditions. A subject's DNA, obtained from a blood sample, sometimes along with DNA samples from other family members, can be analyzed to determine whether the subject is a carrier of conditions such as sickle cell anemia, Tay-Sachs, and cystic fibrosis (CF). Table 1 lists some genetic conditions for which tests are currently available, along with the population thought to be most likely to benefit from screening. In the future, genetic tests will be available for a wide range of genetic conditions or predispositions, such as susceptibility to breast cancer, depression, schizophrenia, and heart disease.

The available screening tests vary in their accuracy and predictive value. Some tests are highly accurate (sensitive and specific) and have a relatively high predictive value. If both partners test positive for the gene associated with the development of Tay-Sachs disease, for example, they have a 25 percent chance of having a profoundly disabled child with a greatly shortened lifespan. Other tests provide much more equivocal information. About one in 25 Americans are carriers of cystic fibrosis (CF), a serious genetic disorder that can result in morbidity and premature death. The most accurate test for cystic fibrosis carrier status will identify about 85 percent of carriers when given to persons from a higher risk ethnic group, white northern Europeans. This means that there will be a significant number of "false negatives," persons who are carriers but who will not be identified in the screening process. In addition, different genetic mutations appear to be related to differing levels of severity in CF (Institute of Medicine, 1994). CF screening thus presents a much more complex decisional matrix: one or both reproductive partners could be carriers of the CF trait even if both test negative; and the most severe form of the illness might not be transmitted to offspring even if both partners test positive. Most expert review panels have rejected the widespread use of CF screening and have instead recommended that CF screening be applied only to persons with a family history of the disorder (Institute of Medicine, 1994). Yet when posed the hypothetical question, most adults are interested in undergoing the CF carrier screening test (Tambor et al., 1994).

The development of CF screening tests demonstrates some important facts about the utility of genetic testing. The HGP will undoubtedly provide reproductive decision makers with highly accurate tests with great predictive value. Increasingly, however, these tests relate to conditions with very low incidence rates. Should potential reproducers undergo screening for conditions of low incidence? The HGP will also lead to genetic tests which, like the early CF tests, provide ambiguous or potentially misleading information about the risk of a genetic disorder because of problems with false negative and false positive results. The actual rate of genetic screening may vary based on a number of factors, including test convenience, test cost, and the predictive value of the test (Tambor et al., 1994). The convenience of testing, combined with a desire to comply with perceived medical authority, can induce persons to undergo genetic screening that is of little value. In one study, for example, many persons were willing to undergo carrier screening for CF even though they were not planning to have children (Tambor et al., 1994).

In part, the utility of genetic testing depends on whether the information gained permits individuals to make choices that are more satisfying than the choices they otherwise would have made in the absence of testing. Individuals who undergo carrier screening and who reliably test negative for some condition are likely to experience a sense of relief and a greater freedom in deciding whether or not to reproduce, though they may suffer from a type of "survivor guilt" (Institute of Medicine, 1994). Individuals who test positive for the genetic condition can use this information in different ways. Where the trait is recessive, they can select a partner who tests negative for the trait or they can bear the 25 percent risk that a child born of a union between two carriers will be affected by the condition. Knowledge of the genetic risk would permit a couple to use either preimplantation or prenatal genetic testing to determine the genetic make-up of their offspring. Once the genetic status of the embryo or fetus is known, individuals can decide whether or not to carry the pregnancy to term. For either dominant or recessive traits, individuals can decide not to reproduce, to adopt, or to use donated gametes for reproduction (Institute of Medicine, 1994).

It might appear, therefore, that testing provides useful knowledge. There are nonetheless significant disadvantages to genetic testing. Initially, of course, persons who find that they are carriers of some genetic condition may develop feelings of negative self-worth. Further, many individuals could feel burdened by the process of making decisions amid substantial uncertainty about outcomes. How are individuals to weigh the probability of having a child with a genetic disorder with the level of disability inherent in the condition against the "disability" of not being conceived at all? These are complex questions, and individuals must be able to chart the course directed by their own value system in a sea of social assumptions and pressures. The general public is largely enthusiastic about the use of genetic screening; those who have undergone screening favor its use, but by a lesser margin (Charo and Rothenberg, 1994).

The Value of Post-Conception Testing

Post-conception testing can occur at various stages. Recent developments permit the use of certain types of genetic screening on preimplantation embryos produced via in vitro fertilization. Some prenatal screening mechanisms, such as chorionic villus sampling (CVS) or the isolation of fetal cells in maternal blood, can be used as early as 9–14 weeks into a pregnancy. Many commonly-used prenatal diagnostic techniques, such as amniocentesis, percutaneous umbilical blood sampling (PUBS), or ultrasound, cannot be used until later in the second trimester of pregnancy. Each of these techniques presents different health risks to the fetus or mother and has a different level of accuracy in correctly identifying genetic problems (Institute of Medicine, 1994).[2]

The likely impact of the HGP on consumer demand for genetic services is difficult to quantify. Prenatal testing is much more common than carrier screening. The relative "popularity" of prenatal screening is based on motivation and contact with medical professionals. A pregnant woman often is motivated by the desire to ensure that the pregnancy "succeeds." The woman is also much more likely to come into contact with health care professionals who will advise prenatal testing in well-defined circumstances, such as where the woman is older than 35 or has a family history of some heritable genetic disorder. Currently, interest in genetic screening is highest among wealthier patients who are aware of a general or specific genetic risk (Charo, 1995). Persons who are poor (and who therefore do not have access to screening) or who are members of racial, religious, or ethnic groups that fear the eugenic implications of screening tend to be under-represented in prenatal testing programs. As the results of the HGP become widely publicized, those able to afford prenatal screening may create a higher demand for a broader range of services.

As with carrier screening, prenatal testing potentially can reveal any one of hundreds of genetic conditions of varying seriousness, from the existence of extra digits to Down's syndrome to neural tube defects (Institute of Medicine, 1994). The women who undergo prenatal screening no longer have the option of not becoming pregnant, of choosing to reproduce using a different combination of gametes, or of pursuing adoption. Instead, women can choose between abortion (if the diagnosis is made early enough in the pregnancy) and carrying the fetus to term. The male partner in the reproductive process has no legal authority to exercise control over the pregnant woman's choice (*Planned Parenthood of Southeastern Pennsylvania v. Casey*, 1992). A prenatal diagnosis of a heritable genetic defect can have an impact on the future reproductive decision making of a couple, but the immediate issue is the appropriate outcome of the current pregnancy. At some point in the future, genetic therapies may make some conditions amenable to treatment.

Several commentators have noted the negative impact of prenatal testing on women's experience of pregnancy. For women at risk for giving birth to genetically disabled children, the period of time between pregnancy and the outcome of testing can become a "tentative pregnancy" (Rothman, 1986). The period between becoming aware of the pregnancy and receiving the test results can be characterized by anxiety and a lack of bonding to the unborn child.

The availability of genetic tests for untreatable conditions carries with it the implicit suggestion that it would be better to abort a fetus with one of these conditions rather than to bring it to term (Lippman, 1993). The assumptions underlying prenatal screening are troubling to those who seek to affirm the inherent value of persons with disabilities (Kaplan, 1993). Those seeking to justify widespread use of prenatal genetic screening often seem to implicitly assume that women will choose to abort fetuses with disabling conditions: "In the values and language of cost-benefit analysis, prenatal testing programs in which fewer than 50% of parents choose to terminate a fetus diagnosed with a genetic disorder are considered to be 'a failure' " (Institute of Medicine, 1994). In fact, many couples notified that their fetus is affected by some types of genetic conditions will continue the pregnancy to term. One study found that "a minority of parents of children with CF (20%) would abort a CF fetus, suggest[ing] that prenatal diagnosis will not lead to a substantial reduction in the number of CF births among this group" (Wertz et al., 1991). There may be a difference, of course, between prospectively reported and actual rates of abortion. In any event, it is clear that the actual abortion rates for other conditions, such as neural tube defects, are far higher (Press and Browner, 1993).

The available information about genetic abnormalities can create substantial amounts of anxiety for potential reproducers, particularly for older women who have been told that their age places their fetuses at greater risk (Lippman, 1993). Prenatal testing can reduce the anxiety for most women who use it. For others, whose fetuses are found to be carrying a disabling trait, prenatal screening will lead to a series of complex and difficult decisions. Prenatal screening will be most useful if and when effective genetic therapies become available; then, health care providers will be able to "treat" rather than just "inform."

Genetic Counseling

The preceding description of the complex informational and value-laden nature of genetic testing suggests that the purveyors of genetic technology will play an important role in determining the use and outcomes of genetic testing. In one study, about 85 percent of women offered alpha-fetoprotein (AFP) screening for neural tube defects accepted testing, even though most of the women did not understand the test or believe that abortion was an appropriate response to a positive test (Press and Browner, 1993). The researchers concluded that the high acceptance rate was based on "how women were informed about the test and what kind of information they were given." Patients agreed to undergo testing because it was viewed as a routine part of medical care that presented no ethical or moral controversies. High rates of acceptance were also related to repeated persuasive contacts with patients who initially refused testing.

This study about real-world genetic counseling is informative because it contrasts with the theory of genetic counseling. Normatively, all agree that genetic counseling is supposed to be informative but "non-directive" (Fletcher and Evans, 1992). In carrier testing, individuals are to be given information about their genetic risk and about the benefits and drawbacks of testing. Post-test counseling is also required, particularly where the individual has tested positive and needs information about the effect of carrier status on his or her ability to reproduce and about the medical and treatment aspects of the underlying genetic disorder. Prenatal testing raises the same issues, with additional problems created because of the individual's need to make a decision about whether to continue the current pregnancy. The couple will need information about the likely medical and psychological implications of the genetic condition, as well as information about available economic or other support systems.

Individuals who are told that they carry some genetically disabling trait or who are told that their fetus is affected are likely to be emotionally vulnerable and confused. The information overload aspects of genetic counseling can exacerbate this problem; one study concluded that "the availability of prenatal diagnosis does not guide attitudes in one direction but rather creates confusion" (Furu et al., 1993). Non-directive counseling attempts to assist the individual or couple in reaching the decision that is compatible with the couple's own value system. While nondirective counseling has been established as the ethical norm, the AFP study discussed above demonstrates some of the difficulties in actual implementation. Other studies indicate, for example, that the professional training of the counselor can make a substantial difference in counseling technique and pregnancy outcomes. Patients of primary-care providers are more likely to receive "directive" counseling than patients of geneticists, and are also more likely to choose abortion (Institutes of Medicine, 1994).

The HGP will probably add another layer of complexity to the genetic counseling process. As more genetic tests become available, more individuals will become the potential genetic "patients." Some of the problems created will be those of training. Far more genetic counselors will need to be trained to deal with a far broader range of genetic conditions. Other problems will arise from the overwhelming nature of the task of explaining to laypersons the genetic risks they confront, the accuracy of available tests, the predictive value of those tests, the heritability of discovered traits, the implications for offspring, and the effectiveness of any available genetic therapy. Providers may feel pressured to give detailed information and to direct patients toward more testing because of the threat of malpractice liability if a parent gives birth to a child with a disabling genetic condition (Charo, 1993). For patients and providers inundated by genetic information, directive genetic counseling may become more "efficient" and therefore more frequent. Individual patient autonomy and the ability to make choices within one's own value system may suffer accordingly.

Governmental Policies Requiring or Limiting Access to Genetic Testing

Mandatory Genetic Testing

The discussion thus far has suggested that the class of potential reproducers provides a relatively large voluntary market for the tools created by the HGP. A variety of factors might nonetheless limit the demand for testing. First, disincentives to testing can be created by the impact of genetic information on an individual's employability or insurability. Second, individuals might avoid testing for conditions for which there are no current treatments. Third, individuals may consider genetic information morally or philosophically irrelevant to their interest in procreating (Tambor et al., 1994; Faden, 1993).

The potential proliferation in the number of genetic tests may lead to the expansion of mandatory governmental screening programs. There are two issues: (1) Are the states or federal government likely to impose widespread or targeted genetic screening programs? and (2) Would such programs be a valid exercise of governmental power?

As to the first question, an examination of state interests and past governmental testing programs yields an equivocal answer. In our federalist system of government, states are more likely than the federal government to pass laws governing the use of genetic testing.[3] States have several different interests in promoting genetic testing. States generally exercise their police powers to promote public health and safety. Genetic screening tests could be viewed as a method of reducing the risk of transmission of a genetic condition from one individual to his or her children. Similarly, states traditionally have exercised their *parens patriae* to protect children from harm, even from harm inflicted by parents. Finally, states could have an economic interest in preventing the transmission of genetic conditions to children because of the risk that the cost of care would eventually be borne by publicly supported health care programs. It is quite important that the current value of testing programs to the state comes almost entirely from encouraging individuals *not* to reproduce. States can "protect" children only by encouraging their non-existence. State testing programs cannot be designed to protect actual future children until effective genetic therapies are developed.

In practice, states have largely disregarded mandatory adult screen ing programs in favor of mandatory or "routine" newborn screening efforts. Only a handful of states have ever required genetic tests for school-aged children or adults; in each of these cases the targeted genetic condition was sickle cell anemia (Institute of Medicine, 1994). Kentucky still arguably permits nonconsensual sickle cell testing: "Every physician examining applicants for a marriage license may obtain an appropriate blood specimen from each applicant [for the purpose of] ascertain[ing] the existence or nonexistence of sickle cell trait or sickle cell disease, or any other genetically transmitted disease which affects hemoglobin" (Ky. Rev. Stat. Ann. 402.320 (1995)). The vast majority of states have relied on voluntary education and testing programs. The Massachusetts statute is typical: "The department of public health shall furnish necessary laboratory and testing facilities for a voluntary screening program for sickle cell anemia or for the sickle cell trait and for such genetically-linked diseases as may from time to time be determined by the commissioner of public health, such as Tay-Sachs disease, Cooley's anemia and hemophilia, which shall be established by each city and town" (Mass. Gen. L. Ann. ch. 76, §15B (1995)).

One could argue that state expansion of mandatory genetic testing programs is unlikely given the absence of widespread mandatory sickle cell or Tay-Sachs testing for adults. It is clear, however, that mandatory testing programs for these conditions are particularly sensitive because the genetic traits are found primarily in African Americans and Jews of Eastern European descent, respectively (Andrews, 1987). Indeed, the history of even a small number of mandatory testing programs primarily targeted to African Americans is a fairly strong statement about either the level of state concern with genetic conditions or the continuing propensity of states to carry out eugenic policies targeted at racial minorities, or both. African Americans and members of other racial or ethnic groups fear that advances in genetics will provide a new opening for discrimination (Bernier, 1994; Nsiah-Jefferson, 1993).

It is possible to look elsewhere for additional evidence of state interest in mandatory testing programs. Initially, genetic screening programs can be analogized to state sponsored pre-marital screening programs for syphilis or gonorrhea. In the 1970s, most states required couples to undergo testing for these sexually transmitted diseases (STDs) before marriage. The theory underlying the testing was simple: Couples seeking to marry were likely to reproduce; these STDs could be transmitted to children before or at birth; and treatment for the STD could reduce the health risk to children. In recent years, many states have repealed their pre-marital testing requirements, in large part because they were not cost-effective. Pre-marital screening tests rarely yielded positive results and failed to address STD transmission outside of marital relationships or in marital relationships after the time of testing (Brandt, 1985). These factors also retarded interest in mandatory pre-marital HIV screening. Only two states, Illinois and Louisiana, enacted such programs and both eventually were repealed (Leonard et al., 1995).

The history of the STD screening programs suggests several hypotheses about prospective genetic screening programs. First, mandatory government screening programs are more likely to arise for relatively common and/or serious genetic conditions. Rarer conditions of greater severity might become a part of a governmental screening program, for example, along with more widespread conditions of lesser severity. Second, the differential treatment of diseases such as syphilis and HIV supports the hypothesis that state interest in testing programs is at least partially dependent on the likelihood that the testing program will eliminate the anticipated harm. Traditional STD testing could directly reduce the rate of STD transmission between partners or to children because of the availability of treatment. The effectiveness of pre-marital HIV screening, in contrast, is attenuated because it depends on behavioral change to prevent transmission, such as by individuals choosing to forgo procreative sexual activity.

Genetic screening programs also have a counterpart in newborn screening programs, many of which implicitly provide information about the genetic characteristics of the newborns' parents (Clayton, 1992). Most states have programs testing for phenylketonuria (PKU) and congenital hypothyroidism; conditions which, if left untreated, can lead to mental retardation. State-sponsored newborn testing programs have expanded, however, to include testing which identifies conditions which either have no current treatment or which are not associated with any known pathology. Much of the screening is mandatory or "routine": parents typically have to "opt-out" of the screening rather than having to give informed consent for the screening to be accomplished (Clayton, 1992). While some have argued that state-sponsored newborn screening programs typically are based on economic concerns rather than on the police power or *parens patriae* (Clayton, 1992), there can be little cost savings to a screening program which detects an untreatable or non-pathological condition. These programs evidence the fact that the state is interested in identifying children with genetic conditions at least in part to influence their parents' future reproductive decision making.

Most recently, public health policies have begun to strongly encourage HIV screening of women who are pregnant or who are considering pregnancy; several states also are considering adding HIV to the required battery of newborn screenings. These trends both support the view that the state is, at least in part, interested in imposing certain types of knowledge on potential reproducers with the goal of influencing future reproductive behavior. The state's interest may be to encourage treatment of HIV-related illnesses for the mother and newborn and to reduce the transmission of HIV from mother to child through the administration of azidothymidine (AZT) (Peckham and Gibb, 1995). But there is more at work here than concern about current health risks and treatment. In the abortion-shy code language of public health authorities, women who are informed that they are HIV-positive can "make informed reproductive decisions," such as to choose abortion or to refrain from future reproduction (U.S. Centers for Disease Control and Prevention, 1995b).

This analysis of other testing programs suggests that governments might be interested in expanding mandatory screening programs, particularly where the tested-for genetic characteristic is somewhat prevalent and has serious consequences. These testing programs are likely to be imposed before conception for two reasons. First, pre-conception programs do not directly implicate the controversial abortion issue. Second, pre-conception testing generally is less physically intrusive and therefore less medically risky than some types of post-conception testing. Of the post-conception testing technologies, those which are less physically intrusive and risky, such as testing fetal cells found in maternal blood and ultrasound, are the most likely to be used in mandatory testing programs.

The next major issue is whether the government has the legal authority to impose testing programs. The federal government has the power to impose public health regulations on states as a precondition for the receipt of federal funding. Under the police power and *parens patriae*, states have the constitutional authority to protect the health and safety of the general public and to provide special protection to children. Would these interests be sufficient to support mandatory screening programs?

Mandatory genetic screening programs raise several constitutional concerns. Although the Supreme Court has never described its dimensions with any clarity, it would appear that individuals have some constitutionally protected liberty interest in controlling their own medical treatment (*Cruzan v. Director, Missouri Dept. of Health*, 1990). The Fourth Amendment also protects individuals from unreasonable searches and seizures, including blood tests. Screening programs focused on particular groups would raise equal protection problems.

An individual's right to control his or her bodily integrity and medical treatment can be outweighed by a compelling state interest. The state can intrude on individual liberties where the intrusion is necessary to serve a compelling state interest in protecting public health. The more intrusive the state policy, the more substantial the justification likely to be required. In *Jacobson v. Massachusetts* (1905), for example, the Supreme Court held that mandatory vaccination policies were a permissible exercise of the state's power to prevent the spread of contagious diseases. A state could argue that its mandatory testing program reduced the rate of "genetic disease" transmission by preventing the birth of persons with pathological genetic conditions. This argument is weak in several respects. First, of course, preventing the birth of an individual is a very different matter from preventing the transmission of a disease to that person. In the absence of effective gene therapies, the state's interest in protecting public health becomes an interest in preventing birth, hardly a traditional interest of the state. Second, it is not clear that mandatory testing programs are "necessary" and "narrowly tailored" even to this objective. Voluntary education and testing might be as effective. Both voluntary and mandatory testing programs suffer from the "defect" that individuals could still choose to reproduce, frustrating the state's goals.

State testing programs are more likely to withstand Fourth Amendment constitutional challenges. To be constitutional, searches must be "reasonable." In the civil context, courts generally will uphold mandatory testing programs where "the invasion of an individual's legitimate privacy interest is outweighed by the governmental interests asserted to justify the search" (Bobinski, 1992). States could argue that a premarital genetic testing program is the virtual equivalent of long-standing pre-marital screening for STDs. In both cases the state seeks to determine whether a health threat exists and to give information to the individual that can be used to reduce the threat. Individuals could argue that STDs are largely treatable, while most genetic conditions currently are not; however, courts are still likely to find the search "reasonable."

States might have an interest in targeting testing programs where a particular genetic condition is unevenly distributed across the population. Yet the selection of some persons for coercive testing raises equal protection concerns. Could states require testing for certain classes of persons? The standard of judicial scrutiny applied to targeted testing programs will depend on the nature of the classification within the program. Race-based classifications will receive the closest judicial scrutiny and will be upheld only when narrowly tailored and necessary to achieve a compelling state interest, such as the interest in protecting public health. Gender-based classifications generally receive a lesser degree of scrutiny by the courts; a screening program which targeted pregnant women might be upheld so long as the gender disparity was necessary to serving an important governmental objective. A testing program applied to all persons seeking to marry (so long as it was not used to prevent marriage) would likely be judged under the rational basis test, the easiest standard for the government to meet. A court merely would have to find that a significant percentage of the class of persons who are contemplating marriage might also be contemplating reproduction.

Thus, the broader the state testing program the more likely it is to be upheld in an equal-protection challenge. State attempts to require the testing of all, however, diminish the economic and logical rationality of testing where the particular genetic condition is primarily found in some groups. The most constitutionally innocuous approach would be to require genetic screening before marriage for persons with a family history of a heritable disability.

Leaving constitutional questions aside, state testing programs might violate the Americans with Disabilities Act (ADA). There are two issues: Are members of the targeted group "individuals with disabilities," and would a program of mandatory testing constitute impermissible "discrimination" under the act? The Equal Employment Opportunity Commission (EEOC) (1995) recently issued interpretive guidelines indicating that when an employer discriminates against individuals who are carriers of disabling genetic traits, the individuals are being regarded as having a disability and they therefore are entitled to protection under the ADA. This definition of "disability" is likely to be carried over to the other parts of the ADA, which prohibit discrimination in public accommodations and public services. The ADA generally also protects persons based on their "association" with a person with disabilities, such as a family relationship. Persons with a family history of genetic disorders are thus likely to be considered disabled for purposes of the public services portion of the act and entitled to protection from discriminatory state actions (Americans with Disabilities Act, 1990).

As to the second issue, there is some controversy about the extent to which the ADA restricts the state's traditional authority to use coercive measures to protect the public health. Under Title II of the ADA, "[N]o qualified individual with a disability shall, by reason of such disability, be excluded from participation in or be denied the benefits of the services, programs, or activities of a public entity, or be subjected to discrimination by any such entity" (ADA, 1990). An individual who presents a "direct threat" to the health or safety of others in the governmental program may not be considered "qualified" (Department of Justice, 1992). This language arguably would not cover a state's effort to protect potential children from being born. More generally, several commentators have argued that Title II's provisions should be used to constrain the state's ability to single out individuals with disabilities for a coercive health measure (Gostin, 1995; cf. Dugan, 1993). In any event, broad-based testing or voluntary testing would appear to present no difficulties under the statute.

States certainly have an interest in promoting the use of genetic screening tests. Whether that interest is expressed in the form of mandatory testing programs will depend on several factors. First, mandatory genetic testing is much more likely to be used and to be found legally permissible when genetic therapies are available to remedy discovered genetic defects. When genetic therapy becomes available, genetic testing will more genuinely fulfill states' interest in protecting health, rather than in merely preventing birth. Second, as an economic matter, mandatory programs are most likely to develop where the underlying condition is serious and the cost of testing, per discovered case, is relatively low. Third, the adoption of mandatory programs will be tied to the political and moral culture of each state. A state with a strong "right to life" lobby, for example, is unlikely to adopt mandatory screening tests which might indirectly encourage abortion.

Given these legal, practical, and political constraints, it is likely that genetic screening programs will remain "voluntary" for the foreseeable future. It is important to recognize, however, that states can still exercise substantial persuasive power even in a voluntary testing scheme. State statutes that require physicians to "offer" genetic testing to persons considering marriage or pregnancy, for example, carry with them the message that such testing is a social, and possibly moral, good (see Press and Browner, 1993). Ultimately, such voluntary testing programs can become a form of coercion, where the availability of a technology carries with it the implicit demand for its use. As philosopher Laura Purdy has noted with respect to other reproductive technologies: "[W]hat start out as new options come to be accepted as the standard of care, which women are not really free to refuse" (Purdy, 1995).

The potential for coercion in state policies requiring that persons be "offered" information also has been demonstrated with respect to state abortion regulations. States seeking to guide women toward choosing pregnancy over abortion have adopted waiting periods and detailed informed consent provisions in which women must be offered information about fetal development. The Supreme Court has held that these statutes further the state's interest in protecting fetal life and that they do not constitute an "undue burden" on a woman's right to choose whether or not to procreate (*Planned Parenthood of Southeastern Pennsylvania v.*

Casey, 1992). Courts could use the same rationale to uphold state laws requiring that pregnant women or persons considering procreation be offered information about genetic testing services.

Prohibiting Genetic Testing

After all this discussion of the state's interest in mandatory screening programs, it may seem contradictory to consider the possibility that states will act to restrict access to genetic testing. Many states currently regulate access to genetic testing by prescribing the qualifications of those eligible to provide genetic testing and counseling services or by establishing genetic screening programs at public health care institutions (Clayton, 1994; see also, California Business and Professional Code §1229 (1995)). A few states have regulated access by prohibiting the use of such tests by insurers or employers (see Ohio Rev. Code Ann. §1742.42 (1995)). Despite this paucity of regulation, it is possible that states might be tempted to limit access to certain types of genetic testing services, either because of the specific type of genetic trait at issue or because of the close connection between genetic testing of pregnant women and abortion.

Preimplantation genetic screening constitutes one area of potential controversy. This genetic screening holds great promise for those who know that they are carriers of disabling genetic conditions because it permits parents to test embryos for the condition before implantation. Embryos with the problematic genetic condition can then be discarded; those without the condition can be implanted (Norton, 1994). This technique, while expensive, permits parents to avoid a potentially more traumatic abortion. For some states, however, the failure to implant an embryo because of genetic factors will be as objectionable as an implantation followed by an abortion. The procedure becomes even more controversial if it is used nontherapeutically, to select for positive genetic traits rather than merely to avoid genetic pathologies.

Currently, the most controversial specific genetic test is used to determine the sex of the fetus. The use of genetic testing is problematic because it is associated with decisions to abort fetuses or to refuse to implant zygotes of the "wrong" sex, most often females. The issue divides those who ordinarily agree on the need to protect individual liberties. For some, sex identification testing is a constitutionally protected aspect of procreative liberty. For others, it perpetuates the subjugation of women by inviting fetal femicide. In India, activists succeeding in obtaining legislation that restricts access to pre-natal sex testing (Boland, 1995). Such legislation is unlikely in the United States for two major reasons. First, there is less social pressure to have only male children in this country. As a consequence, testing for purposes of sex identification will have only a marginal impact on the ratio of male to female births. While the morality of sex-based testing has been debated in this country (Danis, 1995), there is no broad-based support for restricting access to this type of testing. Second, sexism is not the only underlying rationale for sex-identification. Some potential parents are concerned with the possibility of bearing a child with a sex-linked genetic disorder (Jones, 1993).

There is good reason to suspect that state efforts to restrict access to preimplantation genetic screening or to other forms of genetic testing would be found unconstitutional. John Robertson contends, for example, that access to certain types of genetic testing could be considered "part of the liberty interest in procreating or in avoiding procreation, and arguably should receive the same degree of protection" (Robertson, 1994). State legislation limiting access to genetic screening would then be subject to some variation of heightened constitutional scrutiny in the courts (cf. *Planned Parenthood of Southeastern Pennsylvania v. Casey*, 1992). It is unlikely that the state would be able to assert a sufficiently compelling justification for limiting access to information about a potential parent's, embryo's, or fetus' genetic condition.[4]

It is more likely that states will attempt to discourage certain types of genetic screening by refusing to fund educational programs or the genetic tests themselves. These restrictions are likely to be motivated by a desire to reduce abortions. Courts have upheld the refusal of federal and state governments to pay for abortion services. States are permitted to favor pregnancy over abortion by choosing to fund one choice but not the other (*Harris v. McRae*, 1980). Federal- or state-funded health programs are constitutionally entitled to prohibit participating health care providers from providing information relevant to the abortion decision. In *Rust v. Sullivan* (1991), for example, the Supreme Court upheld a federal statute that prohibited recipients of Title X family planning funds from "provid[ing] counseling concerning the use of abortion as a method of family planning or provid[ing] referral for abortion as a method of family planning." The Court held that "[t]he Government can, without violating the Constitution, selectively fund a program to encourage certain activities it believes to be in the public interest, without at the same time funding an alternative program which seeks to deal with the problem another way."

Applying these principles to genetic screening programs, anti-abortion jurisdictions could quite practically limit access to genetic testing services by refusing to pay for them or by refusing to pay for medical training programs designed to educate genetic services providers. Tennessee's statutory framework provides a good example. The state-sponsored genetic services program is intentionally limited to reduce the risk that genetic tests will lead to abortions:

> Induced abortions shall not be regarded as treatment. Therefore, procedures or services designed to search out disorders in unborn children which are not treatable shall not be provided for under this part . . . it being the finding of the general assembly that the use of this program to abort unborn children is against the public policy of the state. (Tennessee, 1994)

A state's refusal to fund certain types of genetic services can make them inaccessible to its citizens, particularly those with low incomes.

This section has demonstrated that state attempts to mandate or to prohibit use of genetic testing services are politically unlikely and legally suspect. The situation could change dramatically, however, as effective genetic therapies are developed. The state's interest in protecting unborn children would become a stronger force that might be found sufficient to support certain limited types of state regulation. In the absence of effective genetic therapies, most governmental regulation of testing is likely to be of the "voluntary" variety. Governmental programs designed to encourage or discourage use of genetic tests may be almost as influential as mandatory programs, but will be relatively invulnerable to legal attack.

Governmental Efforts to
Influence Procreative Choice

This section will analyze the ability of government to influence procreative choice once the genetic status of an individual or fetus is known.[5] State regulations in this area could be motivated by the desire to protect children from being born with a specified genetic condition, by the fear that children with genetic disorders will become public charges, or by a state policy of discouraging abortion. This divergence in state interests is naturally associated with a range of potentially conflicting state policies. Theoretically, states could directly prohibit certain types of reproductive choices for persons who carry defective genes by prohibiting marriage, or requiring sterilization or abortion. In the alternative, states could attempt to discourage certain procreative choices, such as abortion, through direct prohibitions, "education" programs, or funding subsidies. Finally, states may wish to influence the ability of potential parents to "design" children. The scope of permissible state regulation in each of these areas will be explored below.

State Efforts to Prevent Procreation

As the discussion of pre-marital screening programs in the preceding section indicated, states traditionally have associated the status of marriage with a propensity, or at least a predisposition, for reproduction. Theoretically, states might attempt to limit the right to marry for those with disabling heritable genetic conditions. We currently recoil from the possibility, yet for others the possible is real. In China marriage is prohibited for those "diagnosed with diseases that 'may totally or partially deprive the victim of the ability to live independently, that are highly possible to recur in generations to come and that are medically considered inappropriate for reproduction' " (Gewirtz, 1994).

In the United States, however, it is absolutely clear that a state could not attempt to repress procreation by denying persons with genetic conditions the right to marry. In *Loving v. Virginia* (1967), the Supreme Court held that the right to marry was fundamental and could be abridged only by the assertion of a compelling state interest. Even assuming that the state's interest in preventing birth could ever be found to be compelling, a marriage ban would not be narrowly tailored to serve this interest. Marriage is more than procreation; procreation occurs without marriage.

A marriage ban also would violate the public services provisions of the ADA. Utah responded to the threat of AIDS by prohibiting persons with HIV infection from marrying. A federal district court struck down the statute, holding that it violated Title II of the ADA (*T.E.P. & K.J.C. v. Leavitt*, 1993). The same principles would apply here. Persons with disfavored genes would be considered protected from discrimination in gaining access to the right to marry (see Department of Justice, 1992).

Mandatory sterilization programs would more directly meet the state's interest in preventing the birth of children who carry some disfavored constellation of genetic characteristics. We need not look as far as China to find state-sponsored mandatory sterilization programs targeted toward those considered to carry heritable traits thought likely to present a risk to public safety, or to the public purse. Legislatures in the United States first began enacting such statutes in 1907. At the peak of eugenic fever, more than half the states had laws permitting the mandatory sterilization of persons who were "feeble-minded," insane, or "habitual criminals" (Dudziak, 1986).

Initially courts upheld the state's authority to mandate sterilization for selected groups. The Supreme Court considered the constitutionality of a Virginia statute authorizing sterilization of the "feeble-minded" in *Buck v. Bell* (1927). Virginia sought to sterilize Carrie Buck, a resident of the State Colony for Epileptics and Feeble Minded. Both Carrie's mother and Carrie's own daughter were alleged to have been "feeble-minded." Justice Oliver Wendell Holmes, whose famous ability to turn a phrase most infamously haunts him in this case, upheld the sterilization, remarking "Three generations of imbeciles are enough." Justice Holmes never identified the constitutional dimensions of a right not to be sterilized in *Buck*. Instead, he focused on the ability of the state to intrude on individual liberty for its own protection:

> We have seen more than once that the public welfare may call upon the best citizens for their lives. It would be strange if it could not call upon those who already sap the strength of the State for these lesser sacrifices, often not felt to be such by those concerned, in order to prevent our being swamped with incompetence. It is better for all the world, if instead of waiting to execute degenerate offspring for crime, or to let them starve for their imbecility, society can prevent those who are manifestly unfit from continuing their kind. (*Buck v. Bell*, 1927)

The Supreme Court revisited state sterilization statutes in *Skinner v. Oklahoma* (1942). The statute in *Skinner* permitted forced sterilization of repeat criminal offenders. Without explicitly repudiating *Buck v. Bell*, the Court invalidated the statute. *Buck* was not determinative, the Court noted, because its underlying statute applied equally to all. In contrast, the Oklahoma provisions distinguished between apparently similar criminal offenses in the process of identifying those subject to sterilization. Theft of a chicken, the Court noted, could result in sterilization, while embezzlement of the same chicken would not. This statute, then, was unconstitutional under the Equal Protection Clause. Furthermore, the Court noted with some solicitude the nature of the right the state sought to extinguish:

> We are dealing here with legislation which involves one of the basic civil rights of man. Marriage and procreation are fundamental to the very existence and survival of the race. The power to sterilize, if exercised, may have subtle, far-reaching and devastating effects. In evil or reckless hands it can cause races or types which are inimical to the dominant group to wither and disappear. There

is no redemption for the individual whom the law touches. . . . He is forever deprived of a basic liberty. (*Skinner v. Oklahoma*, 1942)

Skinner's suggestion that procreative choice might be a fundamental right for constitutional purposes was echoed in a series of Supreme Court decisions between 1972 and 1992 dealing with contraception and abortion. In each of these cases, whatever their disagreements about abortion, a majority of the Supreme Court indicated that a fundamental right of privacy protected an individual from "unwarranted governmental intrusion into matters so fundamentally affecting a person as the decision whether to bear or beget a child" (*Eisenstadt v. Baird*, 1972; *Planned Parenthood of Southeastern Pennsylvania v. Casey*, 1992). It is likely that the Court would continue to apply strict judicial scrutiny to mandatory sterilization cases, even though it has applied the less stringent "undue burden" test in abortion cases.

Skinner's repudiation of mandatory sterilization policies may have curtailed some sterilization programs, but coercive use of sterilization continued well into the 1970s, despite federal efforts to ensure that sterilizations were truly voluntary (Ehrenreich, 1993). In *Avery v. County of Burke*, for example, the plaintiff charged that the practices of a county board of health and board of social services wrongfully coerced her to undergo sterilization. The minor, a pregnant teenager, was tested and then (erroneously) told that she had sickle cell trait. Thereafter,

[t]he nurses urged her to consider sterilization. They told Avery and her mother that . . . childbirth would either immediately endanger her life or take two or three years off of her life. They cautioned that a woman with sickle cell trait is unable to take birth control pills. One nurse subsequently told Avery and her mother that it would be to their advantage to sign the sterilization consent form. A doctor associated with the clinic also recommended sterilization after warning that pregnant women with sickle cell trait are more susceptible to numerous diseases. Based on these representations, Avery and her mother consented to the sterilization. (*Avery v. County of Burke*, 1981)

The Court of Appeals upheld Avery's right to sue the county for an unconstitutional deprivation of her right to procreative liberty. The court found that the county had a constitutional obligation to ensure that its policies and practices did not lead to coercive sterilizations.

Finally, states theoretically could attempt to prevent procreation by requiring abortion where genetic tests reveal that a fetus has a genetic anomaly. This seems an unlikely event outside horrific feminist science fiction (cf. Atwood, 1987). Optimistically, one could argue that such policies will not be imposed because of our profound respect for reproductive autonomy. The constitutional right to choose to have children once you are pregnant appears to be recognized even by Justice Scalia, who ordinarily is hostile to non-textual constitutional rights (*Planned Parenthood of Southeastern Pennsylvania v. Casey*, 1992). Perhaps more importantly, states will not induce abortions because such a policy would directly conflict with the still-powerful pro-life agenda. Even China's initial policy of requiring abortion of fetuses carrying genetic defects was altered after international criticism. Currently, Chinese "[c]ouples whose unborn children are found to have a serious genetic defect will be consulted by a doctor, who will 'give them medical advice for a termination for the pregnancy' " (Girwirtz, 1994).

From a modern legal perspective, the infirmities of coercive eugenic statutes seem both numerous and painfully clear. They intrude deeply, and sometimes permanently, into the fundamentally protected right of procreative choice. They are vulnerable to equal protection and procedural due process challenges. Finally, they would violate the provisions of the ADA. Nor are the old eugenics statutes redeemed by any compelling, or even rational, state interest. Looking back on the eugenics movement of the early 1900s, it is easy to say that these state policies were simply bad science: persons were subject to mandatory sterilization even when their "conditions" were not scientifically proven to be heritable. Further, the misuse of this bad science became indelibly stained by the mandatory sterilization and extermination programs of Nazi Germany.

For all these reasons, states are quite unlikely to revive mandatory eugenic programs. It is nonetheless still worth retelling the history of the judicial response to these programs, if only as a cautionary tale about the difficulties that our courts then had in identifying what seems so clearly wrong to us now. Furthermore, there are two recent developments that suggest that we may be condemned to repeat history because, as usual, our present facts and circumstances seem different enough to justify a similar response. The two relevant developments are the HGP—which will replace the bad science of the past with "truth"—and the use of voluntary incentive programs—which are more acceptable because they are not mandatory.

The HGP will make it possible for policy makers to distinguish past eugenic policies from current attempts to use knowledge to improve the general welfare. Those seeking to promote "correct" reproductive decisions will be able to point to scientific studies, which presumably will have fewer scientific flaws than those used by eugenicists in the 1920s

(Dudziak, 1986). Policy makers will have access to increasing amounts of information connecting individual genotypes with adverse consequences, some serious.

Government entities are most likely to implement voluntary, rather than mandatory, programs. Two current examples demonstrate the trend. First, states have considered adopting mandatory testing programs as a method of reducing the rate of HIV transmission from woman to child; yet in the end, states have instead implemented "voluntary" or "routine" testing (see, e.g., Anonymous, 1995). The second example appears more distantly related but is nonetheless telling. Policy makers have responded to the perception that women on welfare are having too many children not by forbidding reproduction but by creating financial incentives for reduced childbearing. Thus, current welfare reform proposals typically include benefit caps or the complete denial of benefits for groups of women who have children while on welfare or while they are minors (see, e.g., Paige, 1995).

States might attempt to encourage individuals not to procreate by requiring that genetic services providers give certain types of information to the carriers of some genetic traits. A statute might require, for example, that providers give detailed information about the effect of that trait on unconceived or unborn children (see *Planned Parenthood of Southeastern Pennsylvania v. Casey*, 1992). State efforts to influence people to refrain from reproduction run the risk of coercion even where they are theoretically voluntary. First, the *Avery* case demonstrates the fact that coercion via biased information has occurred in the past. Second, the state's attempt to influence procreative choice can have a powerful effect in shaping social norms about correct behavior. Third, the state's ability to differentially fund procreative choices may, as a practical matter, determine the outcome for low- to moderate-income families. Even "voluntary" programs may ultimately intrude on the ability of people to choose to procreate given a known risk of certainty of passing on a genetic disorder.

Restricting Access to Abortion

Thus far we have focused on the state's interest in restricting reproduction for persons found to carry some disabling genetic condition. Yet in many states, politicians may be as or more interested in preventing persons from aborting fetuses with genetic conditions. In these jurisdictions, the issue will be whether an individual will be able to choose not to carry the pregnancy to term free from state interference.

An individual may obtain information about the potential genetic characteristics of his or her offspring at different stages: before conception, after conception but before implantation, after implantation but early in the pregnancy, or late in the pregnancy. Generally speaking, the technology of genetic testing is permitting genetic assessments at increasingly early stages of pregnancy. It remains true, however, that many women will not discover that their fetus has a genetic condition until later in pregnancy. Under *Roe v. Wade* (1973), the time period of decision making was critical to determining the permissible scope of state interference. Individuals were free to use contraceptive methods to prevent conception and, with respect to in vitro fertilization methods, were free to discard some or all pre-implantation embryos without state interference (cf. *Davis v. Davis*, 1992). After implantation and during the first trimester of pregnancy, the state had little ability to regulate abortion. During the second trimester, when abortion became a more complicated and dangerous medical procedure, the state was permitted to regulate abortion only as necessary to protect the health of the woman undergoing the procedure. Finally, during the third trimester, which the Court equated with the beginning of fetal viability, states were permitted to regulate and even prohibit abortion except where the abortion was necessary to preserve the life or health of the woman.

The plurality opinion in *Planned Parenthood of Southeastern Pennsylvania v. Casey* (1992) retained some degree of constitutional protection for a woman's right to choose abortion but discarded *Roe*'s trimester framework and adopted a less restrictive standard for reviewing the constitutionality of state abortion regulations. One important change wrought by *Casey* is a heightened recognition of the state's interest in promoting fetal life prior to viability. States are permitted to further this interest so long as the state regulation does not impose an "undue burden" on the ability of the woman to choose abortion. This state interest is strong enough, for example, to support state informed consent provisions which mandate that women considering early abortions be given information about abortion and its alternatives so long as the information is "truthful and not misleading" (*Planned Parenthood of Southeastern Pennsylvania v. Casey*, 1992). Women considering abortion because of fetal genetic anomalies might well be able to argue that they should be protected from state informed consent requirements which focus on the development of "normal" fetuses because such information would be untruthful and misleading with respect to their pregnancies. A state would still be able, however, to require that women be given truthful information about the developmental possibilities of their fetus and about the availability of state or private assistance in raising a child with the particular genetic condition (see Charo and Rothenberg, 1994).

The *Casey* plurality retained the point of viability as the time at which the state's interest in fetal life became compelling enough to support substantial restrictions on the woman's right to choose abortion. Echoing *Roe*, the plurality found that such restrictions were permissible so long as abortion was available where necessary to protect the life or health of the affected woman. In practice, states have enacted a wide range of statutes governing abortions after viability. In most states, abortions are restricted to the constitutional limits established in *Roe* and reaffirmed in *Casey* (see, e.g., North Carolina, 1979). Congress is considering a proposal to restrict access to late abortions (Mead, 1995).

Currently, in a few jurisdictions, post-viability abortions are permitted where the fetus has a "severe" or "grave" "abnormality." The important issues in these states are the definitions of "severity" or "gravity" and the identity of the person applying the definition. That is, is the woman, her physician, or some state official to determine whether a particular genetic condition is sufficiently severe? (Charo and Rothenberg, 1994). Each of these states requires one or more physicians to certify that the fetus' condition meets the "severity" test. The Kansas statute is typical:

65-6703. Abortion prohibited when fetus viable, exceptions; penalty.

(a) No person shall perform or induce an abortion when the fetus is viable unless such person is a physician and has a documented referral from another physician not financially associated with the physician performing or inducing the abortion and both physicians determine that: (1) The abortion is necessary to preserve the life of the pregnant woman; or (2) the fetus is affected by a severe or life-threatening deformity or abnormality. (Kansas Statutes Annotated, 1994)

The severe restrictions on post-viability abortions reemphasize the need to make genetic determinations early in pregnancy. To some extent, the legal limits on abortion argue for a very conservative use of genetic testing when the results will be obtained after fetal viability. Genetic testing would seem useful at this stage only if the parents would be able to use the diagnostic information to prepare, psychologically and medically, for the impact of the child's birth.

A few states attempt to prohibit sex selection abortions. (Jones, 1993). The Illinois statute purports to regulate sex-based abortions even prior to viability:

(8) No person shall intentionally perform an abortion with knowledge that the pregnant woman is seeking the abortion solely on account of the sex of the fetus. Nothing in Section 6(8) [720 ILCS

510/6] shall be construed to proscribe the performance of an abortion on account of the sex of the fetus because of a genetic disorder linked to that sex. If the application of Section 6(8) [720 ILCS 510/6] to the period of pregnancy prior to viability is held invalid, then such invalidity shall not affect its application to the period of pregnancy subsequent to viability. (Illinois Compiled Statutes, 1995)

The statute clearly constitutes an "undue burden" on a woman's right to choose abortion prior to viability and would therefore be found unconstitutional under *Casey*. The statute is just as clearly constitutional in its application post-viability, where the Supreme Court permits states to regulate and even prohibit abortions so long as they are available to protect the life and health of the pregnant woman.

This section has reviewed the state's power to limit procreative choice by restricting access to abortion. Practical considerations such as funding and availability will also have an important impact on a woman's ability to choose to abort a fetus. The federal and state governments typically refuse to subsidize abortions, even those based on the genetic condition of the fetus. These policies have been found constitutionally permissible (*Harris v. McRae*, 1980); the absence of funding means that abortions—particularly second trimester abortions—will be unavailable to poor women. In addition, there is a shortage of medical providers willing to perform abortions (Rosenfield, 1994). There are only a few providers in the entire country who will perform late-term abortions because of genetic abnormalities (Mead, 1995). Thus, a woman's ability to choose to abort a fetus with a genetic anomaly will be dependent on governmental regulation, economic factors, and geography.

State Efforts to Regulate Genetic Engineering

The final area of potential state interference in procreative choice is also the most currently fanciful. Suppose that the HGP provides us with not only the ability to identify problematic genes, but also with the technology to affirmatively choose certain genetic characteristics. Loosely, "negative" genetic engineering has come to mean the use of technology to eliminate disabling genes; "positive" genetic engineering means the use of that technology to select particular genetic traits where no genetic abnormality exists (Attanasio, 1986). Positive genetic engineering is considerably more controversial. Should individuals be permitted to engage in either negative or positive genetic engineering free from state interference? The policy arguments are clear, even if the appropriate outcome is not.

On the one hand, negative genetic engineering is the natural outgrowth of the HGP and holds the potential for eliminating many disabling genetic conditions. The technology could facilitate reproduction for those who currently have made the choice not to reproduce because of fear that they will pass on a genetic disability. Even positive genetic engineering seems to fit well within social norms. Potential parents already engage in a primitive form of genetic engineering in exercising choice over mate selection, or, as with gamete donation, by choosing donors with certain characteristics. Genetic engineering would constitute a refinement of the age-old effort to select a mate with characteristics that we value, such as green eyes, intelligence, or kindness. Owen Jones (1993) agrees, arguing that control over one's genetic potential should be considered a core aspect of our constitutionally protected liberty interest in procreation. Jones contends that parents should be permitted to used "Trait-Selection Technologies" so long as "their actions are neither designed to, or in all probability likely to, result in 'clearly and significantly damaging' effects on the future child" (Jones, 1993).

On the other hand, genetic engineering should be avoided because it may either fail or prove too successful. Geneticists agree that the genetic code is complex and that genes associated with one trait also may have effects on other systems or attributes of an individual. Attempts at negative genetic engineering could result in other, unanticipated negative consequences for the child. In a social sense, negative genetic engineering represents a continuation of the devaluation of persons with disabilities (cf. Drimmer, 1993). Positive genetic engineering is also problematic: increasing height, for example, might decrease life span because of negative cardiovascular consequences. Further, widespread adoption of genetic engineering could affect species survival as we blithely select out characteristics with short-term drawbacks that may have long-term evolutionary advantages (Norton, 1994). Say, for example, that individuals prefer to have thin offspring and that genetic engineers identify a gene associated with high metabolic levels and low fat storage. This engineering process may be appropriate so long as there are cheap and stable food supplies. It may be disadvantageous if food supplies become unstable and individuals need to rely on fat storage for survival.

Genetic engineering could be too successful as well. The technology is likely to be available only to the relatively affluent. Affluent families might not only rid themselves of disadvantageous genetic characteristics but also affirmatively select characteristics that promote continued success. If genetic engineering is successful, then it could result in the reification of current patterns of unequal access to income and wealth (Attanasio, 1986).

These conflicts are likely to be played out in several stages and in different arenas. The development of genetic engineering technology might be stifled by funding restrictions or research prohibitions. The federal government has struggled with whether to fund research on fetal tissue (Fletcher and Ryan, 1987). States could ban "experimentation" on fertilized ova. Illinois provides one statutory example: "No person shall sell or experiment upon a fetus produced by the fertilization of a human ovum by a human sperm unless such experimentation is therapeutic to the fetus thereby produced. Intentional violation of this section is a Class A misdemeanor. Nothing in this subsection to prohibit the performance of in vitro fertilization" (Illinois Compiled Statutes, 1995). Even the Illinois ban would permit genetic manipulation of the gametes prior to fertilization.

Government funding restrictions are constitutionally permissible under *Harris v. McRae* (1980). Statutes prohibiting genetic research might merit different constitutional treatment than statutes prohibiting the use of the technologies, once they are developed. Research on genetic manipulation will require the use of real human tissue and, at some point, the birth of genetically engineered children. Parents could argue that a research ban unconstitutionally infringes on their fundamental rights to procreate and to make medical decisions on behalf of their potential children. A state could argue that it has a compelling interest in protecting the to-be-developed fetus from the risks of genetic manipulation. The threat of injury will be great enough at the outset to lend credibility to the state's claim. Courts might, therefore, uphold state efforts to regulate genetic experimentation so long as the regulatory efforts were narrowly tailored to reducing the risk of injury to the conceived fetus.

Paradoxically, states would have a more difficult time prohibiting the use of genetic manipulation once it has been perfected. Once genetic manipulation has been determined to be "safe," then the state's interest in its regulation is reduced. In these circumstances, the rights of the parents to control their own procreative potential and to direct medical care for their unborn child would seem superior to a state's asserted interest in preventing the entrenchment of inequality. Parents generally are permitted to invest whatever monetary resources they can marshall to promote the success of their children. Private school education and investments in home computers provide but two familiar examples. Once genetic manipulation has been proven to be "safe," a state's ability to regulate might be limited to regulations designed to protect the unborn child from affirmative harm. For example, one prominent defender of the right of parents to mold their children's genetic destiny draws the line at parents inflicting "affirmative harm," "such as when deaf parents might seek to create a deaf child" (Jones, 1993).

Conclusion

The HGP will lead to the "geneticization" of much of what we currently think of as our health, talents, and personality. The process of reproduction, which has always been a black box within which our genetic cards are shuffled and dealt out to a new generation, will seem less random and more controllable. In that sense, the HGP presents the possibility of greatly improving the procreative lives of men, women, and their children. These improvements are most likely to come if individuals are able to maintain control over the decision of whether and how to use genetic information and technology. As past eugenic failures indicate, positive reproductive health outcomes are most likely to come from giving potential parents—rather than the state—the power to determine whether or not to make use of the information and tools that the HGP will surely eventually provide (Rothenberg, 1993).

Notes

1. The genetic literature often distinguishes between genetic testing, which is conducted on individuals known to be at risk for carrying some genetic disorder, and genetic screening, which is conducted on groups of individuals not known to be at risk for the condition. For simplicity, this chapter will ignore this technical terminological distinction.

2. In recent years, for example, there has been a significant amount of controversy regarding whether amniocentesis or CVS should be considered the optimal method of obtaining fetal material for genetic testing. Amniocentesis is generally performed later in pregnancy than CVS. The cell culturing and genetic analysis can be performed more quickly for CVS than for amniocentesis. There have been concerns, however, that CVS presented slightly higher risks to the fetus and that a confirmatory amniocentesis test might be necessary in a small percentage of cases (Institute of Medicine, 1994). The most recent studies indicate that amniocentesis performed at 15–18 weeks gestation carries approximately twice the risk of miscarriage as

CVS. CVS, however, presents a risk of transverse limb deficiency not found in amniocentesis, particularly when the CVS is conducted at less than 10 weeks gestation (U.S. Centers for Disease Control and Prevention, 1995a). Choosing between CVS and amniocentesis is merely the first difficult choice in prenatal screening.

3. The federal government does not ordinarily directly regulate to protect public health unless there is a threat that crosses state lines, such as a communicable disease, or a specific medical device or drug that can be used in many states. This does not mean that the federal government is uninterested in health issues; nothing could be further from the truth. What it does mean is that federal regulation in this area is often indirect. Instead of passing a statute which would require all persons to undergo genetic testing, for example, the federal government is much more likely to pass a law which requires that states have in place a specified type of genetic testing program before they can receive federal public health funding. Thus, the National Sickle Cell Anemia Control Act of 1972 offered states financial assistance in establishing sickle cell testing programs, but required that the programs be voluntary (Institute of Medicine, 1994). For this reason, much of the discussion in the remainder of this chapter will focus on the role of the states in regulating the use of genetic testing and technology.

4. The connection between long-standing social prejudice and the availability of genetic testing may be replayed in other areas. The controversial (and yet to be independently verified) study finding a genetic link to male homosexuality provides one example (Hamer et al., 1993). Some gay activists feared that parents would use prenatal screening to selectively abort fetuses "at risk" for homosexuality (Crewdson, 1995). The researcher responded by arguing for the development of ethical or statutory guidelines forbidding such practices (King, 1994).

5. As noted above, most direct regulation in this area is likely to occur at the state rather than federal level of government. The federal government may indirectly regulate by requiring that states have in place certain types of regulation in order to be eligible for federal funding.

References

Americans with Disabilities Act, 42 U.S.C.A. §12132 (West Supp. 1995).

Andrews, Lori B. *Medical Genetics: A Legal Frontier*, 228 (1987).

Anonymous. "New Law Requires AIDS Test to Be Offered in Prenatal Care." *San Francisco Chronicle*, October 14, 1995, A17.

Attanasio, John B. "The Constitutionality of Regulating Human Genetic Engineering: Where Procreative Liberty and Equal Opportunity Collide." University of Chicago Law Review 53:1274 (1986).

Margaret Atwood. *The Handmaid's Tale* (1987).

Avery v. County of Burke, 660 F.2d 111, 113 (4th Cir. 1981).

Bernier, Barbara L. "Class, Race, and Poverty: Medical Technologies and Socio-Political Choices." Harvard Black Letter Journal 11:115–43 (1994).

Bobinski, Mary Anne. "Risk and Rationality: The Centers for Disease Control and the Regulation of HIV-Infected Health Care Workers." St. Louis University Law Journal 36:275 (1992).

Boland, Reed. "Population Policies, Human Rights, and Legal Change." American University Law Review 44:1274–75 (1995).

Brandt, Allan M. *No Magic Bullet: A Social History of Venereal Disease in the United States Since 1880*, 177 (1985).

Buck v. Bell, 274 U.S. 200, 207 (1927).

California Business and Professional Code §1229 (West 1995) (qualifications of persons performing genetic testing under state program).

Charo, R. Alta. "The Human Genome Project and Reproductive Decisionmaking," 19–23 (unpublished contract paper, 1995).

Charo, R. Alta. "Legal and Regulatory Issues Surrounding Carrier Screening." Clinical Obstetrics and Gynecology 36:580–83 (1993).

Charo, R. Alta, and Rothenberg, Karen H. " 'The Good Mother': The Limits of Reproductive Accountability and Genetic Choice," in *Women and Prenatal Testing: Facing the Challenges of Genetic Technology*, 106, 110–11 (1994).

Clayton, Ellen Wright. "Screening and the Treatment of Newborns." Houston Law Review 29: 99, 101–103, 116, 127–28, 145 (1992).

Clayton, Ellen Wright. "What the Law Says about Reproductive Genetic Testing and What It Doesn't," in *Women & Prenatal Testing: Facing the Challenges of Genetic Technology*, 161–66 (Karen H. Rothenberg and Elizabeth J. Thomson, eds.)(1994).

Conner, J. M. and Ferguson-Smith, M. A. *Essential Medical Genetics*, 142 (4th ed. 1993).

Crewdson, John. "Study on 'Gay Gene' Challenged; Author Defends Findings against Allegations." *Chicago Tribune*, June 25, 1995, C1.

Cruzan v. Director, Missouri Dept. of Health, 110 S.Ct. 2841 (1990).

Danis, Jodi. "Recent Development, Sexism and 'The Superfluous Female': Arguments for Regulating Pre-Implantation Sex Selection." Harvard Women's Law Journal 18:219 (1995).

Davis v. Davis, 842 S.W.2d 588 (1992).

Department of Justice, Regulations Implementing ADA Title II, 28 C.F.R. §35.104, §35.130(b)(6), (8), and Pt. 35 Appendix (1992).

Drimmer, Jonathan C. "Cripples, Overcomers, and Civil Rights: Tracing the Evolution of Federal Legislation and Social Policy for People with Disabilities." UCLA Law Review 40:1341–45 (1993).

Dudziak, Mary L. "Oliver Wendell Holmes as a Eugenic Reformer: Rhetoric in the Writing of Constitutional Law." Iowa Law Review 71:843–47 (1986).

Dugan, James C. "Notes, The Conflict Between 'Disabling' and 'Enabling' Paradigms in Law: Sterilization, the Developmentally Disabled, and the Americans with Disabilities Act." Cornell Law Review 78:537–41 (1993).

EEOC, Compliance Manual, volume 2, EEOC Order 915.002, section 902 (1995).

Eisenstadt v. Baird, 405 U.S. 438, 453 (1972).

Ehrenreich, Nancy. "The Colonization of the Womb." Duke Law Journal 43:515 (1993).

Faden, Ruth. "Reproductive Genetic Testing and the Ethics of Parenting." Fetal Diagnosis and Therapy 8(suppl. 1): 142 (1993).

Fletcher, John C., and Evans, Mark I. "Ethics in Reproductive Genetics." Clinical Obstetrics and Gynecology 35:766 (1992).

Fletcher, John C., and Ryan, Kenneth J. "Federal Regulations for Fetal Research: A Case for Reform." Journal of Law, Medicine and Health Care 15:126 (1987).

Furu, T., Kaarlainen, H., Sankila, E.-M, and Norio, R. "Attitudes toward prenatal diagnosis and selective abortion among patients with retinitis pigmentosa or choroidermeia as well as among their relatives." Clinical Genetics 43:164 (1993).

Gewirtz, Daniel S. "Toward a Quality Population: China's Eugenic Sterilization of the Mentally Retarded." New York Law School Journal of International and Comparative Law 15:147–48.

Gostin, Lawrence O. "The Resurgent Tuberculosis Epidemic in the Era of AIDS: Reflections on Public Health, Law, and Society." Md. Law Review 54:1, 92–96 (1995).

Hamer, D. H., Hu, S., Magnuson, V. L., Hu, N. Pattatuccim, A. M. "A Linkage between DNA Markers on the X Chromosome and Male Sexual Orientation." *Science*, 261:321 (1993).

Harman, Christopher R. *Invasive Fetal Testing and Treatment*, 124 (1995)(table 1).

Harris v. McRae, 448 U.S. 297 (1980).

Illinois Compiled Statutes, 720 ILCS 510/6 (7), (8) (West Smith-Hurd's 1995).

Institute of Medicine, Committee on Assessing Genetic Risks. *Assessing Genetic Risks: Implications for Health and Social Policy*, 41, 72–73, 74, 75–82, 147–68, 153 (Lori B. Andrews, Jane E. Fullarton, Neil A. Holtzman, and Arno G. Motulsky, eds. 1994).

Jacobson v. Massachusetts, 197 U.S. 11 (1905).

Jones, Owen D. "Reproductive Autonomy and Evolutionary Biology: A Regulatory Framework for Trait-Selection Technologies." American Journal of Law & Medicine, 19: 195, 197, 223 (1993).

Kansas Statutes Annotated §65-6703 (1994).

Kaplan, Deborah. "Prenatal Screening and Its Impact on Persons with Disabilities." Clinical Obstetrics and Gynecology, 36:610–611 (1993).

Kentucky Revised Statutes Annotated §402.320 (1995).

King, Warren. "The Science of Sexuality." *Seattle Times*, October 18, 1994, A10.

Leonard, Arthur S., Bobinski, Mary Anne, Closen, Michael L., Hermann, Donald H. J., Isaacman, Scott H., Jarvis, Robert M., Rivera, Rhonda R.,

Schultz, Gene P., and Wojcik, Mark E. *AIDS Law and Policy: Cases and Materials*, 96 (1995).

Lippman, Abby. "Prenatal Genetic Testing and Geneticization: Mother Matters for All." Fetal Diagnostic Therapy, 8(suppl 1):181, 183 (1993).

Loving v. Virginia, 388 U.S. 1 (1967).

Maddalena, Anne, Bick, David P., and Schulman, Joseph D. *Molecular Diagnosis of Genetic Disease*, 37:437 (1992).

Massachusetts General Laws Annotated, ch. 76, §15B (1995).

Mead, M'Evie. Editorial, "Late-Term Abortion Curbs Are Hazardous." *St. Louis Post-Dispatch*, July 24, 1995, 7B.

North Carolina, Opinion of Attorney General to Mr. Lewis H. Nelson, M.D., Assistant Professor, Bowman Gray School of Medicine, 48 N.C.A.G. 136 (1979) (no lawful abortion after 22 weeks based on abnormality or limited life-span of fetus).

Norton, Vicki G. Comment, "Unnatural Selection: Nontherapeutic Preimplantation Genetic Screening and Proposed Regulation." UCLA Law Review 41:1581, 1582–83, 1611–13 (1994).

Nsiah-Jefferson, Laurie. "Access to Reproductive Genetic Services for Low-Income Women and Women of Color." Fetal Diagnostic Therapy 8 (suppl. 1):121 (1993).

Ohio Revised Code Annotated §1742.42 (1995) (temporary statute prohibiting mandatory genetic screening by HMOs).

Paige, Connie. "Law Rips Weld-fare; Sparks Fly over Cuts for Teen-age Mothers." *Boston Herald*, October 13, 1995 p. 1.

Peckham, Catherine, and Gibb, Diana. "Mother-to-Child Transmission of the Human Immunodeficiency Virus." New England Journal of Medicine 333:301 (1995).

Planned Parenthood of Southeastern Pennsylvania v. Casey, 112 S.Ct. 2791, 2807, 2821, 2823–24, 2874 n.1 (1992).

Press, Nancy Anne, and Browner, C. H. " 'Collective Fictions': Similarities in Reasons for Accepting Maternal Serum Alpha-Fetoprotein Screening among Women of Diverse Ethnic and Social Class Backgrounds." Fetal Diagnosis and Therapy 8 (suppl 1):97, 105–106 (1993).

Purdy, Laura M. "*Children of Choice*: Whose Children? At What Cost?" Washington & Lee Law Review 52:203, 207 (1995).

Robertson, John A. *Children of Choice: Freedom and the New Reproductive Technologies*, 33 (Princeton: Princeton University Press, 1994).

Rosenfield, Allan. Editorial, "The Difficult Issue of Second-Trimester Abortion." New England Journal of Medicine 331:324–25 (1994).

Rothenberg, Karen H. "The Law's Response to Reproductive Genetic Testing: Questioning Assumptions about Choice, Causation and Control." Fetal Diagnosis and Therapy 8 (suppl 1): 163 (1993).

Rothman, Barbara Katz. *The Tentative Pregnancy: Prenatal Diagnosis and the Future of Motherhood* (1986).

Rust v. Sullivan, 111 S.Ct. 1759, 1763, 1771 (1991).

Skinner v. Oklahoma, 316 U.S. 535, 540 (1942).

Tambor, Ellen S., Bernhardt, Barbara A., Chase, Gary A., Faden, Ruth R., Geller, Gail, Hofman, Karen J., and Holztman, Neil A. "Offering Cystic Fibrosis Carrier Screening to an HMO Population: Factors Associated with Utilization." American Journal of Human Genetics 55:626, 634–35 (1994).

T.E.P. & K.J.C. v. Leavitt, 840 F. Supp. 110 (1993).

Tennessee Code Annotated 68-5-504(a)(2) (1994).

United States Centers for Disease Control and Prevention. "Chorionic Villus Sampling and Amniocentesis: Recommendations for Prenatal Counseling." MMWR 44 (No. RR-9):10–11 (1995a).

United States Centers for Disease Control and Prevention. "Recommendations for Human Immunodeficiency Virus Counseling and Voluntary Testing for Pregnant Women." MMWR 44 (No. RR-7):6 (1995b).

Wertz, Dorothy C., Rosenfield, Janet M., Janes, Sally R. and Erbe, Richard W. "Attitudes toward Abortion among Parents of Children with Cystic Fibrosis." American Journal of Public Health 81:995 (1991).

Six

Access to the Genome and Federal Entitlement Programs

Maxwell J. Mehlman

The Human Genome Project (HGP)—the massive research initiative to map and sequence the human genome—will produce a host of potential benefits and detriments for individuals. Most of the work on the ethical, legal, and social implications of the project has focused on the potential detriments—for example, the use of genetic information to block access to employment and to restrict the availability of private health insurance. This chapter focuses instead on the potential benefits from the HGP, and specifically, on the role of federal health care entitlement programs, chiefly Medicaid and Medicare, in providing access to these benefits.

The potential benefits from the HGP fall into three categories. The first is information about an individual's genetic endowment. When the mapping and sequencing of the genome is completed, a complete map of the human genome will have been created. By analyzing a sample of one's own DNA (or the DNA of one's offspring) and comparing the results with the master printout, an individual is likely to be able to identify the individual's (or the individual's offspring's) predisposition to genetically related diseases and conditions, as well as the extent to which the individual possesses desirable, genetically based physical and mental characteristics. While this information can harm the individual if it is used improperly or if it falls into the wrong hands, it can allow the individual to make welfare-enhancing choices about reproduction, life-style, and health care needs to prevent or minimize future harms or to plan for their occurrence.

The second category of benefits is interventions to prevent and treat genetic disorders. These modalities include alternative reproductive technologies, such as in vitro fertilization, symptomatic and ameliorative treatments for expressed disorders that are produced with genetic engineering techniques such as recombinant DNA, and ultimately both somatic and germ cell genetic therapy. The genetic engineering techniques of recombinant DNA and gene splicing are already available and are being applied extensively in the manufacture of pharmaceuticals and other products for human use and to alter the genetic make-up of plants and other animals. Gene therapy in humans is underway on an experimental basis, with investigations being conducted or planned in children with severe combined immunodeficiency syndrome, patients with metastatic melanoma and homozygous familial hypercholesterolemia, and HIV-infected patients with non-Hodgkin's lymphoma.[1]

The final type of benefit from the HGP is the ability to produce or enhance desirable physical and mental characteristics. This includes the use of exogenous agents, such as human growth hormone, "positive eugenics," such as selective fertilization, and ultimately genetic engineering to alter an individual's genetic endowment. Once the human genome is mapped, we will know the location not only of the genes responsible for genetic diseases and disorders, but of those associated with all other genetically related traits. When the nucleotides that make up these genes have been sequenced, the same gene-altering techniques may be employed to affect these traits as well.

The potential significance of access to these benefits cannot be underestimated. This is particularly true of genetic therapy and enhancement techniques. Individuals with access to genetic therapy will be able to avoid or to reduce the personal and economic impact of genetic illnesses and disorders, ranging from poor eyesight and dentition to cancer and heart disease. Depending on which traits turn out to be genetically related, individuals with access to genetic enhancements will be able to make themselves or their offspring taller, stronger, more attractive, more resilient to illness and stress, more intelligent, and perhaps longer lived. Access to genetic therapy and enhancement will mean no less than the ability to redefine the individual's degree of social and economic opportunity.

Given the expected demand for these services, the impact of the HGP on federal entitlement programs will be profound. To understand why, it is necessary to appreciate the nature and role of these programs.

The Nature of Federal
Entitlement Programs

There are four major federal entitlement programs or "FEPs": Medicare, Medicaid, the health care programs of the Veterans Administration, and CHAMPUS, which covers health care for civilian employees and dependents of the military. If some version of health care reform is enacted, the role of the federal government will increase, although it is not clear exactly how this would take place. Such a development would make the following discussion even more important, because it would enlarge the pool of potential claimants to entitlements to genetic services. The discussion that follows, however, will focus merely on Medicare and Medicaid; between them, they currently distribute approximately 27 percent of all health care benefits in the United States.[2]

The purpose of Medicare and Medicaid is to provide access to health care. Medicare is a program primarily for the elderly, although it also provides services to individuals who are permanently disabled and to people with end-stage renal disease. Persons who qualify for Medicare are covered regardless of their financial means. Medicaid is a joint federal-state program that provides health care services to certain persons who are poor, chiefly to those who qualify for Aid to Families with Dependent Children (AFDC). Together, these programs provide access to the needy elderly who cannot pay for health care themselves (directly or through private insurance), or—in the case of the well-to-do elderly— to persons who society has decided should not have to pay.

In the process, these programs redistribute wealth. Medicare is financed by a tax on wages. While most Medicare enrollees paid this tax themselves when they were working, health care for the elderly is subsidized by younger workers; the program is so expensive that it takes the taxes of four current workers to finance the benefits for one current recipient.[3] Medicaid is financed by general federal and state tax revenues, with the federal government paying up to 83 percent of the costs of the state programs, depending on the per capita income of the state. In essence, persons earning enough to pay taxes subsidize those who are poor and unemployed.

The Effect of the HGP on the
Demand for Genetic Services

The HGP will dramatically increase demand for genetic services within FEPs. The elderly will seek information about their predisposition to the genetically related diseases of old age and genetic therapy to prevent or ameliorate the effects. They will also press for somatic cell interventions to retard the aging process itself. Medicaid recipients of childbearing age will seek information about the genetic endowments of their potential offspring and interventions to prevent disorders or to produce desirable traits. In addition, they will demand prognostic information and therapy for themselves and their families.

The impact of the increased demand for genetic services on the costs of FEPs is unclear. Certainly, obtaining, interpreting, and explaining genetic information will be expensive. These costs, however, may be offset by the reduction in health care expenditures associated with more accurate diagnosis and treatment and the prevention of genetic disorders. Gene therapy itself is likely to be extremely costly, particularly when the techniques are first developed. Long-term program costs may be reduced, however, with savings from the elimination of chronic genetic illnesses. On the other hand, by preventing diseases or conditions that would have resulted in early death, gene therapy may increase the costs of care for nongenetically-related health problems in those who live longer. Genetic enhancement is also likely to be expensive, and is not likely to reduce program costs.

Any attempt to estimate whether program costs as a whole will increase or decrease as a result of the HGP is highly speculative, but it can be assumed that, at least in the short run—that is, before savings from reduced future illness, if any, are realized—the effect will be to increase substantially the demand for cost-increasing services. To the extent these services are covered, therefore, the effect will be to put significant upward pressure on program costs.

The prospect of increased demand for genetic services leading to increased costs for FEPs raises two key issues: To what extent will FEPs provide access to these benefits, and to the extent that this increases program costs, how will the increased costs be financed?

To begin to answer these questions, it is necessary to understand how these programs currently provide access to health care services. Access to services under both Medicare and Medicaid is contingent on four factors: eligibility, copayment, coverage, and availability.

Limits on Access under Current Programs

As noted earlier, Medicare provides services only to (1) persons 65 and over, plus (2) persons who qualify for disability payments under the Social Security Disability Income program (individuals who are permantly disabled) and (3) persons with end-stage renal disease. Medicaid eligibility is more complicated. In general, persons whose income is below the federal poverty level and who either are eligible for AFDC or who are aged, blind, or disabled may enroll in the program, although the states may establish income thresholds below the federal poverty level, and usually do. Combining the requirements of the two programs, large segments of the population are ineligible for benefits: primarily single, nondisabled adults and childless couples below the age of 65.

In order to receive benefits under Medicare, eligible individuals must pay a portion of the costs themselves. Persons receiving benefits under Part A, which principally covers inpatient hospital care, must pay an annual deductible ($696 for 1994) and a portion of costs once the patient exceeds a certain annual number of days of hospitalization (60 days in 1994). Persons who choose to enroll in Part B, which covers physician care, must pay a monthly premium ($41.10 in 1994), an annual deductable ($100 in 1994) plus 20 percent of the fees set by Medicare. In addition, physicians who do not agree to accept the Medicare fee as payment-in-full may require an extra payment from their patients. Copayment is less prevalent under Medicaid, although some states require patients to pay a nominal sum for prescription drugs. Finally, Medicare establishes lifetime limits on the number of days of hospitalization it will pay for an individual; once the limit is exceeded, such as in the case of a chronic illness requiring lengthy hospitalization, the patient must bear the entire cost of care. This limit was removed under the Medicare Catastrophic Coverage Act of 1988, but restored when that act was repealed in 1989.

Beyond restrictions on access imposed by eligibility and copayment requirements, both Medicare and Medicaid categorically deny coverage for certain services. Both programs exclude services that are experimental, as well as routine dental and eye care. Medicare excludes long-term care. Medicaid denies coverage for abortions, and allows states to refuse to cover certain non-experimental organ transplants, such as liver transplants. In addition, the prospective payment system used by Medicare and many state Medicaid programs prohibits hospital admissions for certain procedures that can be performed on an outpatient basis, and through its payment formulas and external oversight mechanisms, restricts the length of stay of those patients who are admitted.

The most far-reaching effort to restrict coverage under federal entitlement programs is the Oregon Medicaid Demonstration Project. A public commission categorized all health services into 709 "condition-treatment" pairs, and the state legislature mandated that the state Medicaid program cover only 587 of them.[4] Among the services that would not be covered are breast reconstruction after mastectomies (not currently covered by the Oregon Medicaid program), treatments for psoriasis, bone marrow transplants for non-Hodgkin's lymphoma, and viral pneumonia in infants.[5] The quid pro quo for these limits on coverage is that the state will enlarge the population eligible for Medicaid to include all persons whose incomes fall below the federal poverty level.[6] Because both the coverage limits and the expansion of eligibility would violate federal law, the state petitioned the Department of Health and Human Services for a waiver from the conflicting provisions of the law. While the Bush administration rejected the request on the ground that the Oregon plan violated the Americans with Disabilities Act, the Clinton administration approved the waiver, subject to certain conditions pertaining to disability-related issues.[7]

The final factor bearing on access under FEPs is the availability or supply of services. Some geographic locations, particularly rural areas, lack tertiary care facilities and high-technology equipment such as magnetic resonance imaging machines.[8] In addition, the relatively low levels of reimbursement under Medicaid reduce the number of physicians and other providers willing to treat Medicaid beneficiaries. This is particularly a problem with regard to prenatal and obstetrical care.

Trends in Access

To predict how FEPs are likely to cope with the demand for genetic services that will result from the HGP, we can examine how these programs are reacting to pressures to increase access, on the one hand, and to reduce health care spending on the other.

One way or another, limits on access due to the inability to meet eligibility criteria are bound to disappear. Whether the approach that eventually is taken will be to expand eligibility under the FEPs themselves, or to create new governmental entitlement programs, or to mandate that individuals be covered under private insurance, is unclear. It is safe to say, however, that by the time that the HGP has begun to stimulate demand for genetic services to a significant degree, all persons in the United States will be entitled to some form of government-mandated third-party payment for health care.

At the same time that it faces pressures to expand eligibility, however, the government also is being called upon to reduce national health care expenditures. The movement to expand third-party payment programs removes a common method of reducing spending: limiting access by restricting eligibility. To stem budget increases, for example, state Medicaid programs traditionally have lowered income thresholds in order to exclude persons who would otherwise be eligible. Prior to the increase in eligibility to cover all persons with incomes below the federal poverty level, or FPL, for example, the Oregon Medicaid program only provided benefits to persons who qualified for AFDC if their incomes fell below 58 percent of the FPL.

Even if the federal government mandates universal health insurance, it might impose eligibility restrictions under future FEPs. For example, if Medicare and Medicaid were retained and government-subsidized private health insurance were provided for those who were not covered by FEPs or insured by their employers, a means test might be added to the eligibility criteria for Medicare, with those persons over 65 who had incomes or assets above the means threshold relegated to purchasing private insurance with their own funds. So long as the nation remained committed to providing universal access to health care, however, this would merely shift costs from government to private programs rather than lowering overall spending. Therefore, the government will need to pursue other methods in order to curtail health care costs.

Undoubtedly, the federal government will attempt to reduce prices for health care, and it will be aided in doing so by the increased leverage it will have as a result of the expansion of eligibility under government programs. However, price controls alone are unlikely to be able to curtail spending in the face of increased demand for services, particularly for genetic services stemming from the HGP. The government will continue to feel strong pressure to restrict access to health care generally, and to new, expensive genetic services in particular. Having lost the ability to restrict access by limiting eligibility, the government will be left instead with the options of copayment, and restrictions on coverage and/or availability.

Maintaining or increasing the amounts that individuals pay for health care under government programs might be one way of limiting access to the genetic services that will emerge from the HGP. Those persons who could not afford the copayments would not receive services, even though they were technically "eligible" for benefits. Medicare in particular has increased copayments as a means to help control program costs. For example, the annual deductible under Part A of Medicare has grown from $492 in 1986 to $696 in 1994. Furthermore, the most recent effort to *reduce* copayments under Medicare—the Medicare Catastrophic Coverage Act—failed miserably when Congress repealed the law under pressure from those elderly persons who would have footed the bill.

Copayments represent fairly obvious limitations on access, however. In a nation committed to universal access, they are likely to be increasingly unacceptable as a cost-containment approach.

The same is true of overt restrictions on availability, or supply, particularly those that affect specific geographic areas or minority populations. For example, the government is likely to be under political pressure to increase the number of physicians and facilities for rural and inner-city residents. Yet shortages are likely to be an inevitable result of efforts to control costs, particularly if prices for health care are forced down substantially. Hospitals may be unwilling to purchase new technologies if their revenues are reduced, and health care professionals may refuse to treat patients who cannot supplement third-party reimbursement from their own resources. The government might try to force unwilling providers to treat patients, but it is unclear if it could do so successfully, or what the effect would be, for example, on the number of physicians entering or remaining in the market.

Furthermore, the government may be tempted to foster shortages deliberately as a method to contain costs, particularly if it can rationalize its behavior as something other than overt rationing. For example, the government might assert that it was merely encouraging "regionalization" or volume-based "centers of excellence" for certain high-technology services. This technique appears to be employed by national health systems such as Canada's, for example, where widespread queuing, at least for elective services, is reported.[9] Whether deliberate or not, therefore, limitations on access as a result of the unavailability of services are likely to persist.

The final approach to limiting access is to restrict coverage. Faced with budget shortfalls, the government might well insist that it is unable to provide access under FEPs to specific services, particularly to the new, cost-increasing technologies emerging from the HGP.

While Medicare law precludes coverage for certain categories of services such as dental, eye, and nursing home care, as noted earlier, the Medicare program historically has defined the scope of covered services very broadly. The law itself stipulates that, with the exception of the categorical exclusions, beneficiaries are entitled to all items and services that are "reasonable and necessary for the diagnosis or treatment of illness or injury or to improve the functioning of a malformed body part."[10] This has been interpreted to preclude the government from refusing to pay for care on the ground that it is too expensive. In 1989 the Health Care Financing Administration (HCFA) proposed to allow Medicare to refuse to cover a technology if it was not "cost effective"— that is, if it yielded no greater net benefit than a cheaper alternative.[11] This proposal has triggered intense opposition, and was never finalized. In any event, such a regulation would have little impact on new, cost-increasing technologies for which there were no alternatives, which is likely to be characteristic of many genetic services emerging from the HGP.

As a result of the scope of coverage embodied in the statutory language, it has been difficult for the government to limit coverage of specific technologies under Medicare in order to achieve cost savings. The government has had some success in controlling costs by limiting the amount of time patients can remain in the hospital. The average length of stay for Medicare patients declined 17 percent between 1983 and 1986.[12] Restrictions on length of stay alone do not discourage access to specific technologies, however, and would be of little use in restricting access to new genetic services.

The primary method by which the government has limited access to new technologies under Medicare has been to deem them "experimental." For many years, for example, Medicare refused to pay for heart transplants on the ground that their safety and efficacy had not been adequately demonstrated, and that therefore they had not been shown to be "reasonable and necessary." Medicare finally agreed to cover the transplants in 1979, but only if they were performed at the Stanford Medical Center.[13] This policy lasted only nine months, at which time the HCFA revoked Stanford's authorization on the basis that the government lacked adequate data on the success and long-term implications of transplant technology.[14] It was not until 1990 that Medicare once again agreed to reimburse for heart transplants, but then only under strict criteria limiting both the hospitals that could perform the procedure and the patients who could be selected.[15]

The technologies emerging from the HGP initially will be experimental, and it will be some time before Medicare can be expected to reimburse providers for them. How much time it will take will depend on the significance of the expected benefit from the technology, the ratio of benefits to risks, and the degree of demand from both patients and health care professionals. Recent experience with AIDS drugs suggests that the government can be forced to accelerate the transition from experimental to therapeutic (and reimbursable) status given enough public clamor. This is likely to be the pattern for genetic services that promise to prevent or ameliorate serious genetic disorders.

Even after the safety and efficacy of a technology has been demonstrated, the government may delay paying for it on the basis that it remains experimental when the real reason is to hold down costs. For example, it is widely believed that the government has continued to maintain that heart transplants and certain other new technologies are experimental in large part in order to contain program costs.[16] The government might be expected to resist paying for expensive, new genetic services under Medicare for the same reason.

Coverage restrictions under Medicare that limited access to genetic services on the basis of cost are not likely to survive for long, however. The elder lobby is too powerful, and its political power is growing as the population continues to age. Coincidentally, the post–World War II baby boom generation will become eligible for Medicare at approximately the same time that the HGP is expected to be completed. Even if younger voters somehow acquired the ability to thwart the interests of the elderly, they may be unwilling to restrict access to services that they may someday need themselves.

In contrast to Medicare, the Medicaid program is much more likely to restrict coverage of expensive, new technologies. A trend in this direction already is apparent. Until 1988 federal law required state Medicaid programs to provide liver transplants in order to receive federal matching funds. Coverage for these procedures became optional in 1988,[17] and many states have since refused to reimburse for them. The Oregon demonstration project is even more far-ranging. As described earlier, it has created a list of health services ranked on the basis of importance, and denies coverage for all services below an arbitrary cut-off chosen by the state legislature on the basis of budgetary constraints. The Oregon effort has become the spearhead of a growing effort to contract the scope of high technology health care benefits for the poor.

Several factors explain why the trend for Medicaid is so different from Medicare. First, the law underlying the Medicaid program is less clear-cut than the Medicare statute in terms of what services must be provided. There is no statutory language for Medicaid comparable to the "reasonable and necessary" standard under Medicare. Although courts generally have engrafted the Medicare standard onto Medicaid,[18] they have shown some willingness to allow states to deny coverage for services because of their cost.[19]

A second reason that Medicaid is likely to restrict coverage is the growth of the program as a proportion of state budgets. State Medicaid funding increased 10 percent from 1988 to 1989, and almost 17 percent from 1989 to 1990.[20] Medicaid now accounts for almost 14 percent of state budgets nationwide.[21] State budgetary woes have convinced the middle class that the only alternative to increasing taxes is to decrease the scope of benefits provided under Medicaid and other programs for the poor.

In contrast to the growing political dominance of elder Americans, the political power of the poor is weak. While everyone eventually hopes to be eligible for Medicare, most middle- and upper-class taxpayers never expect to be eligible for Medicaid, and therefore have no incentive to retain a generous coverage policy many consider to be contrary to their own self-interest.

Finally, coverage restrictions under Medicaid have been rationalized on the basis that they forestall cuts in eligibility. As noted earlier, the customary method for trimming Medicaid budgets has been to disqualify individuals from being entitled to any benefits, such as by lowering income thresholds. Limited coverage would seem preferable to none at all. Going a step farther, the Oregon project has justified its coverage limits on the basis that they allow the state to *expand* Medicaid eligibility, and to provide benefits, albeit incomplete, to all persons whose incomes are below the federal poverty level.

In summary, if current trends continue eligibility under FEPs is likely to increase, with more individuals entitled to receive benefits. To hold down costs, the government may try to increase the proportion that individuals must pay for their own care, and to promote "health planning" measures that limit the availability of services in certain geographic areas, but these efforts will be constrained by political pressures aimed at assuring access to some level of health care for all citizens. The most promising approach for limiting health care spending at the same time that eligibility restrictions are relaxed is to deny coverage under FEPs for certain technologies, particularly those that are new and expensive, and particularly for politically weak patient populations such as the poor.

Impact of Access Trends on
Access to Genetic Services

If current trends in access under FEPs persist, the effect will be to deny access to certain genetic services emerging from the HGP for certain populations. One factor that will determine whether individuals are or are not given access will be the nature of the genetic service. Access is likely to vary depending on whether the genetic service being sought is an information service, a genetic therapy, or a genetic enhancement.

A number of forces will combine to pressure the federal government to provide access to information about an individual's genetic endowment. One source of pressure will be the individuals themselves. Many people will seek genetic information so that they can incorporate it into their decisions about health care, lifestyle, reproductive choices, employment, and so on. Access to this information also will be sought by third-party payers, employers, life insurers, and others with a financial stake in the individual's health, productivity, and longevity. Finally, health care providers are likely to press for FEPs to cover the costs of obtaining genetic information.

The HGP will give rise to a new health care industry that decodes an individual's genetic make-up. These entrepreneurs will lobby for FEPs to cover their services so that they can obtain government reimbursement. Health care professionals also will want the government to pay for genetic information so that they can reduce their risk of malpractice for negligent genetic counseling or for failing to obtain their patients' informed consent to treatment. For example, the family of a child born with a genetic disorder might sue the providers of prenatal care on the basis that they failed to ascertain and disclose the risk, thereby precluding the family from preventing or terminating the pregnancy or from attempting to correct the disorder *in utero*. Similarly, a patient might allege that he or she was not given sufficient information about the risks or benefits of a proposed course of treatment or the alternatives because the physician did not obtain and disclose information about the patient's susceptibility to genetic disorders or complications that could affect the outcome. In both cases, the provider would avoid liability if he or she ensured that the patient was given access to genetic information, which would be facilitated by having the information paid for by FEPs.

On the other hand, some individuals will not want access to genetic information about themselves, preferring to remain unburdened by the probability of future harms resulting from their genetic make-up. People also will fear that this information will be detrimental to them if it is obtained by third parties, who will use it to deny them health insurance, employment, life insurance, and the like. These concerns will lead to efforts to restrict access to genetic information on the ground of privacy.

In the end, the degree of access to genetic information provided under FEPs is likely to depend on a combination of factors, including the cost, the funds available for the programs, competing demands for coverage, and whether concerns about privacy are perceived to outweigh the benefits that the information would provide.

FEPs will be under a great deal of pressure to provide access to genetic therapy. The reluctance that some people feel about "playing God" will be overcome by the ability to prevent or ameliorate the suffering from genetic disorders. Assuming that genetic therapy is expensive, the primary impediment to providing widespread access under FEPs will be the cost. This will lead the government to seek ways to limit its coverage of genetic therapy. Initially, reimbursement will be denied on the basis that the technology is experimental. When the technology becomes sufficiently established that this position can no longer be maintained, the government will resort to other approaches. One would be simply to deny coverage on the basis of cost. While this might succeed under Medicaid for reasons discussed earlier, it would only be lawful under Medicare if Congress repealed the statutory requirement that the program cover all "reasonable and necessary" items and services. This would be difficult to accomplish because of the political power of the Medicare constituency.

Another approach would be for society to redefine the distinction between genetic "normality" and "disorder." The notion of normality could be expanded so that many conditions formerly regarded as disorders would no longer be deemed to warrant treatment or prevention. Alternatively, genetic endowments could be reformulated as a continuum, with no clear demarcation between "healthy" and "diseased" states. This would leave the government free to decide not to cover certain therapies, depending on budgetary considerations or on some ordering of priorities similar to the system employed in Oregon.

Assuming that cost constraints lead FEPs to deny coverage for some forms of genetic therapy, one possibility is that these therapies will never be developed. If the government makes clear in advance what types of technologies it will and will not pay for, and if FEPs control an increasing portion of the health care market, it might be assumed that the medical research-and-development community would refrain from investing in these technologies because they would not yield a sufficient return on investment. This assumption is unrealistic, however. In the first place, as I have argued elsewhere,[22] medical research by its nature is not highly responsive to this sort of downstream perspective. Moreover, the basic techniques of genetic therapy are likely to be similar regardless of the specific genetic disease or condition that is targeted, and the mapping-and-sequencing portion of the HGP will reveal the precise location of all human genes. Assuming that FEPs cover genetic therapy for some disorders, it will be impossible to avoid being able to treat most of the others.

If FEPs nevertheless denied coverage for certain genetic therapies, these modalities would be available, but only to persons with more generous health insurance plans, or to those who could pay for the treatments without third-party reimbursement. Because these therapies will be expensive and insurance coverage is not likely to be cheap, only those who are relatively wealthy would have access to them.

The exception is abortion. It is a preventive genetic therapy: it prevents genetic disorders, in the sense that it prevents an individual with the disorder from being born. Furthermore, it is relatively inexpensive, particularly if performed early in pregnancy. If more costly types of genetic interventions were unavailable because they were not covered by FEPs, abortion would become the poor person's gene therapy.

A policy of not covering non-abortion genetic therapies under FEPs increases the demand for abortions. Conversely, the broader the coverage of non-abortion therapies, the less the demand for abortions. Ironically, Congress presently forbids Medicaid—the principal FEP that serves the population that would seek abortions—from funding them. Whether this embargo will persist as other types of genetic therapy become available only to those who can afford them, or whether abortion foes will prevail upon the government to fund the other types of therapy as alternatives to abortion, remains to be seen.

The degree to which FEPs cover genetic therapies may also affect whether individuals are given access to genetic information. If the government refuses to make genetic therapies available under FEPs, it may attempt to deny access to the information that would lead an individual to demand the therapies. For example, it is widely believed that physicians in the United Kingdom do not reveal the potential benefits of kidney dialysis to patients who are not eligible for the treatment under the national health system because of their age and who cannot afford to purchase it in the private sector.[23] Similarly, opponents of abortion may prevent FEPs from providing genetic information about fetal genetic endowments to pregnant women so that they do not seek abortions to avoid bearing children with genetic disorders. This approach is suggested by the recently rescinded federal regulation that prohibited Medicaid providers from furnishing information about abortions to their patients.[24] The constitutionality of this regulation has been upheld by the Supreme Court in *Rust v. Sullivan*.[25]

The alternative of refusing to provide information about noncovered services was rejected by the legislature in Oregon when it enacted the Oregon Medicaid Demonstration Project. One section of the enabling legislation specifically requires physicians to inform patients about services "that are medically necessary but not covered."[26] But the FEP need not actually prohibit providers from informing patients about their genetic endowments. It could simply refuse to provide coverage for the testing necessary to produce the information, which would achieve the same effect with regard to those persons eligible for benefits but unable to afford the costs of testing themselves.

The final category of genetic services is genetic enhancements: interventions that improve an individual's genetic endowment which already is considered to be within a "normal" range. If current policies persist, FEPs are certain to deny coverage for these genetic services. For example, neither Medicare nor Medicaid typically pays for cosmetic surgery.[27] These services will be available only through the private market—to those able to afford them.

Social Consequences

The HGP will create an array of genetic technologies with immense power and promise. Individuals with access to these technologies will be able to stave off disease, increase their life spans, and ultimately refashion their genetic endowments to optimize their social opportunity.

If current access trends continue, many of these benefits will be unavailable under FEPs. Cost constraints will lead to restrictions on the coverage of expensive, new genetic therapies. Genetic enhancements will be withheld on the basis of the government's long-standing unwillingness to pay for services that are deemed unnecessary for "the diagnosis or treatment of illness or injury or to improve the functioning of a malformed body part."[28] At the same time that these genetic services will be excluded from coverage under FEPs, they will be available in the private market to those who can afford them.

The impact on society of this disparity will be unprecedented. Especially if opposition to abortion does not abate, those without access to genetic therapies will have no choice but to continue to endure the burdens of genetically-related diseases, disorders, and death. The population will become sharply divided between those who are "healthy" by virtue of genetic interventions and those who are genetically diseased and impaired.

The impact of unequal access to genetic enhancements will be even greater. Genetically enhanced individuals will gain overwhelming advantages over the non-enhanced. Equal opportunity will disappear. Beyond a narrow range of less desirable social roles and rewards, upward mobility for those without access to enhancement services will become a thing of the past.

The result could be to create a society divided between those with access to the genome and a genetic underclass whose members, except when they escape through rare instances of intermarriage, remain permanently enslaved to their genetic endowments. As more and more advances in genetic therapy and enhancement techniques take place, the differences between the two groups will widen. Eventually, the degree of disparity will dwarf the social distinctions that characterized feudalism, the caste system in India, and even human slavery.

Apart from the question of whether this result is morally tolerable, it is doubtful that current political structures could survive such a social transformation. Those without access to genetic services will struggle to obtain them. Given the stakes involved, the potential for civil strife will be extreme. Forms of government based on notions of freedom and equal rights will be replaced by repressive regimes whose objective is to protect the genetically well-off and to suppress the underclass. Peace and stability will give way to constant rebellion and brutal repression.

The question is whether, anticipating this outcome, society can avoid it. The HGP has just gotten underway, and even the most optimistic researchers do not expect genetic therapy or enhancement technologies to be available to a significant degree for another 15 to 20 years. Yet the consequences of this scientific endeavor are potentially so disastrous, and the remedies so elusive and difficult to implement, that the process of anticipating all of the potential consequences must begin immediately and in earnest.

Alternatives

One way to prevent the foregoing scenario from taking place would be to prohibit anyone from employing genetic therapy or enhancement techniques. A precedent for such a policy is the voluntary ban on recombinant DNA research that was in effect from 1974 until 1975,[29] and the prohibition against the use of fetal tissue in transplant research which was in effect from 1989-1993.[30] Human genetic engineering is likely to offend religious groups and others opposed to the idea of "playing God." These groups may pressure the federal government to refuse to fund research on these techniques. The government could also penalize the use of human genetic engineering by disqualifying the researcher and his or her institution from receiving future federal funding and by imposing criminal sanctions. Even if the government did not officially prohibit genetic engineering, publicity and pressure by opponents could deter research, development, and availability in much the same way that opposition to abortion stalled RU-486 from being marketed in the United States.

Given the disease prevention and therapeutic potential of gene therapy, this approach is unlikely to be adopted or, if adopted, to succeed. Victims of genetic diseases and disorders will insist that research on genetic therapy continue and that the techniques be made available to them. Even if gene therapy were officially banned in the United States, it is likely to flourish in the black market or to be available abroad.[31]

An alternative along the same lines would be to halt the HGP and to forbid its resumption. If no further work were done on mapping and sequencing the human genome, progress in developing genetic therapy and enhancement techniques would be slowed, and even if the techniques themselves were perfected, the absence of a complete genetic landscape would preclude them from being extensively applied. Again, however, the momentum of the project and its potential health benefits are likely to be too great to allow it to be abandoned.

Given that the HGP and the development of genetic therapy are bound to proceed, some of the negative consequences of unequal access to genetic services might be avoided if genetic therapy were allowed, but not genetic enhancement. Nevertheless, the techniques for therapy and enhancement, particularly in germ cells, are likely to be so similar, and the demand so great, that it would be virtually impossible to enforce such a ban. In any event, as the HGP unfolds it may prove increasingly difficult to define a "normal" range of genetic endowments so that "disorders" meriting therapy can be distinguished from "traits" requiring enhancement.

If the development of genetic therapy and enhancement techniques is inevitable, one way to avoid the creation of a genetic underclass would be to expand coverage and eligibility under FEPs to make the technologies universally available. To reduce the price, the government might regard these technologies as public services and regulate their providers as public utilities. Due to the degree of federal research funding, the government might appropriate the patent rights on the resulting products and license their distribution to promote widespread access. However, while these steps might drive down prices and increase access, the costs of these therapies are likely to remain so high that it would be extremely difficult to make them available to all.

The only remaining alternative would be to distribute their benefits equally. One approach would be to regard all genetic differences as creating "suspect classes" under the Constitution and to treat access to genetic technologies as a "fundamental right." This would make it unconstitutional for the government to discriminate against anyone in providing genetic benefits under FEPs on the basis of the individual's genetic endowment without a "compelling state interest," a standard that the government would have difficulty in meeting under most circumstances. Another approach would be a system of genetic "handicapping" whereby individuals with less desirable genetic endowments were given preferences in obtaining access to genetic services under FEPs. Neither of these approaches would entirely avoid the problems of unequal distribution. So long as the government was unable to provide universal access to all genetic services, and services that were not provided under

FEPs were available through the private market, some individuals would have access to benefits that others were denied, and any effort to prevent this would divert resources from providing genetic benefits to enforcing a "war on drugs"–type ban on black-market activity. As uninviting as this scenario appears, a public commitment to equal access, together with the extensive governmental distribution and policing efforts that would be required, may be the minimum condition necessary to avert societal disaster.

Conclusion

The objective of this chapter was to address the benefits or "goods" that can be expected from the HGP, rather than to focus on the "bads," and to explore how these benefits could be distributed through public programs. In the end, however, it has revealed that, by creating a sharply divided society of genetic "haves" and "have nots," even the supposed benefits can become highly destructive.

Yet benefits they remain. The promise that they hold of a better life for those afflicted with genetic diseases and disorders cannot be minimized or avoided. In the relatively few years before these technologies become fully realized, the task is to redefine the scope of entitlements under government programs and the way these programs are financed so that society can obtain the maximum amount of benefit from the HGP with the least amount of harm.

Notes

1. See "Gene Therapy Trials Expand into the Heartland," *AMA News*, March 2, 1992, 3.
2. K. Levit, M. Freeland, and D. Waldo, *National Health Care Spending Trends: 1988*, 9 Health Affairs, 171–74 (1990).
3. Annual Report of the Board of Trustees of the Federal Hospital Insurance Trust Fund, 102d Cong., 1st Sess. (1990).
4. See U.S. Congress, Office of Technology Assessment, Evaluation of the Oregon Medicaid Proposal 1-8 (1992) (hereinafter "*OTA Oregon Report*").
5. Ibid., 5–30, tables 5-11, 5-12.
6. See generally, Mehlman, *The Oregon Medicaid Plan: Is It Just?* 1 Health Matrix, 175–99 (1991).
7. Letter from William Toby, Jr., Acting Administrator, Health Care Financing Administration, to Kevin W. Concannon, Director, Oregon Depart-

ment of Human Resources (Mar. 19, 1993) (on file with the National Legal Center).

8. U.S. Congress, Office of Technology Assessment, *Health Care in Rural America*, 114 (1990).

9. See, e.g., E. Haislmaier, *Northern Discomfort: The Ills of the Canadian Health System*, Policy Review 32 (Fall 1991).

10. 42 U.S.C. §1395y(a)(1)(A). The statute in fact prohibits Medicare from paying for items or services that are not "reasonable and necessary," but the language has been interpreted as defining the scope of entitlements under the program.

11. See 54 Fed. Reg. 4302 (1989).

12. See S. Guterman et al., *The First Three Years of Medicare Prospective Payments: An Overview*, 9 Health Care Financing Review, 67–77 (1988).

13. See 45 Fed. Reg. 52,296 (1980).

14. Ibid., 52,297.

15. See 52 Fed. Reg. 10935 (1987).

16. See generally, J. Katz and A. Capron, *Catastrophic Diseases: Who Decides What?* 168 (1975).

17. See Health Care Financing Administration, *State Medicaid Manual*, 4-203 (1988).

18. See e.g., *Beal v. Doe*, 432 U.S. 438, 444 (1977) ("serious statutory questions might be presented if a state Medicaid plan excluded necessary medical treatment from its coverage").

19. See, e.g., *Ellis by Ellis v. Patterson*, 859 F.2d 52, 55 (8th Cir. 1988) (permitting states to deny coverage of organ transplants as "exotic surgeries which, while they may be the individual patient's only hope for survival, would also have a small chance of success and carry an enormous price tag").

20. *OTA Oregon Report, supra* 7, n.4.

21. Ibid.

22. See Mehlman, "Age-Based Rationing and Technological Development," 33 St. Louis University Law Journal 676 (1989); Mehlman, "Health Care Cost Containment and Medical Technology: A Critique of Waste Theory," 36 Case Western Reserve Law Rev. 778, 840 (1986).

23. See H. Aaron and W. Schwartz, *The Painful Prescription: Rationing Hospital Care*, 101 (1984).

24. Public Health Service, *Standards of Compliance for Abortion Related Services in Family Planning Service Projects*, 58 F. R. 7462. Washington, DC: U.S. Dept. of Health and Human Services; February 5, 1993. 42 C.F.R. §59.

25. See *Rust v. Sullivan*, 111 S. Ct. 1759 (1991).

26. Oregon Senate Bill 27, sec. 6(7) (codified at Ore. Revised Stat. §414.725(7)).

27. See 42 U.S.C. §1395y(a)(10) (Medicare exclusion); see, e.g., *Morris v. Williams*, 67 Cal. 2d 733, 433 P.2d 697, 63 Cal. Rptr. 689 (1967) (California Medicaid program exclusion).

28. See note 10 and accompanying text.

29. See Annas, *Mapping the Human Genome and the Meaning of Monster Mythology*, 39 Emory Law Journal 629, 652 (1990).

30. See M. Specter, "HHS Will Extend Ban on Fetal-Tissue Research," *Washington Post*, Nov. 2, 1989, A3.

31. See D. Callahan, *Setting Limits: Medical Goals in an Aging Society*, 199 (1987) (black market arises if desired health care is outlawed).

Seven

The Implications of the Human Genome Project for Access to Health Insurance

Deborah A. Stone

The Human Genome Project does not augur well for the current system of health insurance in the United States. We have a patchwork combination of public programs and private contracts, all built on deep ideological commitments to preserving competition between insurers for market share and autonomy of employers in deciding upon fringe benefits. In such a system, everybody has an incentive to avoid sick people. And since insurance is a contract to pay for future needs or claims, predictive information about people's likelihood of getting sick turns out to be key.

Predictive medical tests—tests that predict a disease someone might get rather than confirming one they already have—are an old feature of medical practice, of employer hiring practices, and of the insurance enterprise. Genetic information may hold a special fascination in our collective imagination, but its use in and impact on health insurance will be only a change in degree from the status quo, not a fundamental transformation. New information yielded by the Human Genome Project is problematic, I would argue, not because of anything new in the character of this information, or even the scale, but rather because of the institutional context of health insurance into which the results of the Human Genome Project will flow.

The key feature of the institutional context is the splintering of the health insurance market since the mid-1970s, and the consequent erosion of risk-pooling. The institutions of health insurance—commercial, nonprofit, and government carriers, as well as self-insured employers—are less capable of mixing low-risk and high-risk people together in the same pool, and so of spreading the costs of illness among members of a large community. The result is that over 35 million people are relatively permanently uninsured for medical care,[1] an estimated 60 million are uninsured for two months or more during any 18-month period,[2] and untold millions are "underinsured," meaning that their health insurance does not cover much of the care they need.

The major concern about information generated by the Human Genome Project is that it will be used by insurers to further segment insurance pools into smaller, more homogeneous groups, creaming off people who are likely to remain healthy, and leaving the public sector to care for the sick and potentially sick. Thus, in a situation where the nation's health insurance mechanisms are already failing to an important degree, the availability of genetic information about individuals will only hasten the disintegration.

Many analyses of this problem to date have centered on whether and how much insurers and employers actually perform genetic diagnostic testing, and their intentions to perform genetic testing in the future.[3] The two major insurance trade associations, the American Council of Life Insurance and the Health Insurance Association of America, emphasize that no insurer currently uses genetic tests, and that insurers will be cautious about adopting genetic tests because of their expense and low predictive value.

> No insurer—life or health—currently requires genetic tests. One simple and practical reason is cost. . . . Above all, it cannot be emphasized enough that insurers are not using genetic tests in risk assessment, nor are there any plans to do so.[4]

At the same time, the industry has announced its intention to use genetic information the same way it uses other predictive medical information, and defends the economic necessity and fairness of doing so.[5]

Many health policy makers, insurance advocates, and social reformers concerned about both health insurance availability and the ethical implications of the Human Genome Project have called for bans on the use of genetic test information by insurers. These proposals take many forms, including state legislation to prohibit the use of genetic information by insurers, a temporary moratorium on the use, and federal legislation to restrict the use of genetic information by insurers.

Much of this discussion, this chapter argues, is misdirected. First, whether insurers and employers actually perform genetic tests is almost irrelevant to the problem of health insurance access, because they do and will have virtually unlimited access to the information from genetic tests performed in the medical sphere. Second, bans and moratoria on insurers' use of genetic information are unlikely to be effective without addressing the entire structure of health insurance underwriting, benefit design, risk-pooling, and marketing.

Why Insurers Want Genetic Information

Insurers generally give three reasons why they need access to predictive medical information, including genetic test results: fiscal solvency, profit, and fairness.[6] Because they bear the financial risk for the contingencies they insure, insurers need to predict how much money to collect in order to cover their expected payouts. (Insofar as insurers are public agencies, such as Medicaid, they have other sources of revenue besides policy holder premiums; private commercial insurers are limited to premiums and the investment income from premiums and reserves.) Whether they are public, commercial, or nonprofit, insurers need to remain solvent in order to make good on the claims or liabilities represented by their policyholders. Commercial insurers seek to make a profit in addition to being able to pay claims fully. Thus, the purpose of risk classification is to allow insurers "to exercise their right to earn a reasonable profit, and [to provide] an equitable insurance system to policy holders."[7]

Insurers, like any business, have many ways of influencing the balance between revenues and costs. For example, they might seek to trim their administrative costs, to monitor claims more closely, or to control payments to medical care providers more aggressively. One strategy that stands out as extremely important, however, is to *select policyholders who are relatively healthy* and therefore unlikely to incur high medical costs in the future. If an insurer can know in advance that a group is likely to be healthier than average, the insurer can offer a group package at a lower-than-average price, and thus gain a competitive advantage over other insurers.

To use this strategy, an insurer must acquire information about applicants to help predict their likely future claims, and then either reject those with unusually high expected costs or charge them higher prices. This selection strategy is most readily available to commercial insurers. Public programs, though they do select their clientele, must do so according to eligibility rules established in enabling legislation and administrative regulations; nonprofits, such as Blue Cross Blue Shield, are constrained to some extent by their charters and state laws, although they, too, can and do use some risk selection and differential pricing according to risk.

Insurers, especially commercial insurers, see themselves engaged in a strategic game with consumers in which both sides are taking a gamble about expected future costs. (In public programs such as Medicare, Medicaid, or the Veterans Administration system, clients are made eligible relatively automatically and so do not self-select into the programs. People over 65, for example, are not allowed to decline membership in Medicare, even if they think they are extremely healthy or wealthy and will not need medical insurance.) Success in this game requires having more or better (or at least equal) predictive information about future costs than the other side.

There is a widespread, if not universal, perception in the industry that people are more likely to buy insurance when they know they will have occasion to need it. A typical expression of this view is:

> There is a *natural tendency* on the part of the consuming public who need [health insurance] coverage to seek it only when there is a perceived need for medical care, and to cancel the insurance when the immediate need no longer exists.[8] (Emphasis added)

Given this perception of consumers, insurers want to use any information that enhances their ability to predict the need for costly medical care, whenever the information is available to the would-be purchasers of insurance. They want, as the ubiquitous insurance metaphor would put it, "a level playing-field," where they have the same access to predictive medical information as the buyers of insurance. Otherwise, insurers will be "selected against," meaning that people who have taken medical tests and/or know they are at high risk for disease will be highly motivated to purchase insurance and to conceal their condition from the insurer. "Select, or be selected against," goes the old adage taught to every beginning student of insurance.[9] Insurers call this phenomenon "adverse selection." Although there is precious little empirical information on actual consumer behavior in insurance markets, insurers are profoundly influenced by this belief that consumers have a "natural tendency" to buy insurance after they learn of some adverse medical condition.

The fear of adverse selection drives insurers' decisions about whether to acquire and use medical information. One early report of the American Council of Life Insurers explained why insurers would want access to prior genetic testing results *even* if they might prefer not to order genetic tests themselves:

> If test results were unavailable to insurers, applicants who already knew from tests performed by their own physician that they were predisposed to illness or early death could buy large amounts of insurance coverage . . . at rates that do not properly reflect their known risk. If a large number of such applicants bought insurance, or if large amounts of insurance were purchased, the ensuing claims would markedly exceed projected losses.[10]

From an insurer's point of view, the more genetic testing is used in clinical and preventive medicine, the greater the possibility for adverse selection and therefore the more insurers' need to acquire genetic information themselves. This logic is played out vividly in another section of the same report.[11] People who undergo genetic testing and receive negative results, according to the report, will be less inclined to buy health insurance than they might have been without testing, while people who receive positive results will be more inclined to buy. Therefore, the greater the scope of genetic testing in normal medical practice, the greater the proportion of all insurance applicants who will be motivated by knowledge of their higher risk. In a situation where genetic testing has become widespread, if an insurer had no information about the genetic characteristics of its applicant pool and continued to assume the standard mortality or morbidity risks, it would find itself with excess mortality and morbidity, and a resulting imbalance between premium intake and claims payouts.

If insurers feel threatened by potential adverse selection with respect to some disease and are unable to obtain good predictive information, they are likely to use proxy information, even if its predictive value is not very accurate. When California banned the use of HIV antibody tests in health and life insurance underwriting in 1985–86, insurers tested applicants with the T-cell test instead.[12] They used the T-cell test, knowing it was much less specific for AIDS, because to them, avoiding a few infected policy holders was more important than losing sales to a larger number of noninfected people. Similarly, before the advent of good HIV-antibody tests (and to some extent, even afterwards), some insurers used homosexuality as a proxy measure for risk of AIDS, even though that was an extremely crude measure.[13] Some companies took the proxy concept one step further, and used zip codes of residential areas thought to have high concentrations of gays, as well as stereotypically gay occupations, as proxies for risk of AIDS.[14]

Insurers also think that extensive medical underwriting leads to fairness in the allocation of medical care costs. The insurer's definition of fairness is that "each insured [person] will pay in accordance with the quality of his risk."[15] Unfairness occurs when "equal risks are treated differently and/or unequal risks are treated equally."[16] An insurer treats its policyholders fairly when it "establish[es] premiums at a level consistent with the risk represented by each individual policyholder."[17] To do this, insurers must assess each policyholder's risk as accurately as possible, and medical information is the best way to assess the risk.

This definition of fairness is tantamount to saying that ideally, each person should pay for the costs he or she generates, and that cross-subsidy—or healthy people paying for sick people—is unfair. If we had perfect predictive medical information, in this logic, each person *would* pay exactly the cost of his or her own medical care. Of course, self-payment would no longer be insurance, because insurance is by definition risk-pooling, and that is what makes it different from individual savings accounts. Nevertheless, to understand why insurers want to use genetic information, it is crucial to understand the concept of fairness they are pursuing.

How Insurers Acquire Medical Information

Insurers select policyholders through a process of examining applicants called underwriting. Not to be confused with the conventional meaning of underwriting as providing financial backing, the term as used by insurers means the *selection of risks*, or the decision about whom to insure and at what rates. In this sense, the term *underwriting* might better be understood as "close examination." When insurers say they underwrite a certain class of health insurance (such as small group policies), they do not mean they accept all comers in that class, but rather that they subject applicants in that class to a process of individual scrutiny that is not applied to applicants in other classes. In life and health insurance, most of the information insurers need to predict future mortality or morbidity is medical information, and so most of the underwriting is *medical underwriting*. (Insurers also collect information on an applicant's occupation, avocations, and financial situation, for example.) For life insurance, insurers are primarily interested in factors that might lead to a premature death, and for health insurance, they are interested in factors that might indicate a greater-than-average use of expensive medical care.

Although insurers are quick to assure the public that no insurer is currently doing genetic testing,[18] we need to distinguish between *performing the tests* and *using the information* generated by them. Insurers often do perform their own laboratory testing of blood and urine samples in the course of medical underwriting, but their own testing is by far the least important source of medical information on applicants.[19] The vast bulk of information comes from applicants and their medical records. If genetic test results are part of the knowledge of applicants or part of their medical records, the results would be available to insurers. Insurers' access to individuals' medical histories is so extensive that as soon as genetic tests enter into medical practice—even if they are performed only in high-technology centers and not in routine medical practice—the results will be available to underwriters.

Medical Information Provided by the Applicant

Whenever insurance is medically underwritten, the application form asks applicants for medical information about themselves, and often about close blood relatives as well. Typical family history questions ask whether an applicant's parents have had specific diseases, whether either parent died early (e.g., before age 60), and if so, of what cause. Family medical history questions are the most obvious source of genetic information. As one insurance medical director noted, "insurance companies already use genetic data. . . . *To some extent, one might consider family history data a proxy for more specific confirmatory genetic tests.*"[20] If states were to write legislation or regulations prohibiting insurers' use of genetic test results in underwriting decisions, insurers would be likely to use cruder family history information as a proxy. Judging from a common industry claim that use of genetic tests in underwriting would actually increase access to health insurance, many insurers apparently already do use family history information in this way:

> Consider applicants with a family history of Huntington's Disease who have no manifestations themselves. Without genetic testing, no one would know whether these people have inherited the disease. *They would be considered risks that it would be very difficult to insure at reasonably low rates.* But if a genetic test indicated that they were not carrying the Huntington's disease gene, then insurance coverage could be offered at favorable rates.[21]

Most application forms ask whether the applicant has had or has been treated for a variety of medical conditions. If applicants answer yes to any of the health history questions, they are asked to provide more detail. While such medical information is used for all kinds of nongenetic medical conditions, genetic information is and would be caught in this net as well. One medical director evocatively terms this mode of acquiring genetic information "a systems review for footprints of genetic conditions."[22]

Insurers have several ways of inducing applicants to make a full disclosure of their medical conditions and histories. First, all applications require the applicant to sign a statement to the effect that the insurance will not be valid if the applicant has not fully disclosed true answers to the questions. For example, a typical form reads:

> The proposed insured declares that to the best of his (her) knowledge and belief the above answers and statements are complete and true. . . . The undersigned agrees that . . . no insurance shall take effect . . . unless the answers and statements in each part of this application continue to be complete and true as of the date of delivery. . . .[23]

These clauses refer to the insurer's right of recision, the right to deny payment or cancel the insurance within a specified time if the insurer can prove that the policyholder misrepresented or withheld information on the application. Such clauses are invoked often, and could be one vehicle by which insurers could seek not to pay for treatment of genetic diseases.

Another way insurers might obtain genetic information is with more general questions on the application about diseases that have not yet been treated or even manifested themselves. Typical questions ask whether applicants or family members have any "indication" of any disease not disclosed in other questions, whether they have ever been advised to have special examinations, tests, or consultations, and even whether they have ever "discussed" testing or treatments not yet performed. A person who had a positive result for some genetic disease, even one that was only partially genetically determined, or someone who had been merely advised about the possibility of genetic testing would have to disclose that information or risk being denied coverage later.

Physicians' Medical Records

Whenever applicants answer that they have seen a doctor for some problem, they are asked for more detailed information about the problem, as well as the name and address of the treating physician or hospital. Even if an applicant answered "no" to all the questions about specific medical problems, life and health insurance applications typically contain a more general question that will almost always elicit the name of a physician: the forms ask whether the applicant has been hospitalized or seen by a physician in the last five years and request the names and addresses of all treating physicians and hospitals during that period.

All applications require the applicant to authorize the insurer to obtain medical information about the applicant from a wide variety of sources, including physicians, other medical practitioners, hospitals, clinics, other medical facilities, insurance companies, and sometimes employers. In addition, applicants must grant the insurer permission to seek information from any "organization, institution, or person that has any records or knowledge" of their health.

Insurers may request what is known as an Attending Physician's Statement or copies of complete medical records from these physicians and other medical sources. The typical form for an attending physician statement asks the doctor to fill in specific information, but insurers very often ask for copies of complete medical records as well. Significantly, regardless of how insurers *ask* for information, most physicians delegate the completion of these forms to their office staff, and many, if not most, *simply send copies of the medical record*. Photocopying the record is far easier and less time-consuming than abstracting from it. Few physicians are willing to take the time to dictate a special letter or narrative summary for individual insurance requests.[24]

From the medical records, insurers have access to a wide range of information that might not be on the application. Typically, a physician's record includes a family medical history completed at the patient's first visit. Since the norms of primary care practice emphasize prevention through early identification of people at risk for disease, the whole climate of medical practice encourages an expansive disclosure of personal and family medical history. Patients, moreover, are more inclined to give an inclusive medical history and disclose family medical information to physicians (e.g., family histories of cancer, heart disease, or hereditary disease) if they believe that providing the information could help the physician monitor them and prevent disease. Thus, even if an insurer did not ask family history questions on an application, and even if insurers were forbidden to ask questions about family history of genetic diseases, they might still have access to this information via the applicant's medical records.

In addition to family medical history, an applicant's medical records will contain information about diagnostic tests, referrals to specialists, and reports from specialists back to the referring physician, *including any genetic testing or counseling* that has been recommended or performed. Physicians may be very careful to send out only their own notes, and not copies of reports from other physicians, but there is growing evidence that insurers will sometimes take the mere fact of a specialist consultation or the mere ordering of a diagnostic test as evidence of high risk. For example, an insurer excluded coverage of eye disease from a child's health insurance policy, because her mother had once taken her to an ophthalmologist to have her eyes checked, although there turned out to be no problem.[25]

These examples suggest the flavor of the strategic game that insurers are playing. Because the underwriting process is dominated by the fear of adverse selection, insurers are looking for any hint that applicants might know they have a costly disease. Similarly, because expensive illnesses are costly for insurers, they try to use medical records to screen out people who are at high risk for costly diseases. It is easy to see how insurers, in such a mindset, are likely to take the ordering of a diagnostic test, a referral to a specialist, or a visit to a specialist as evidence that the patient or doctor knows something troubling.

Often, medical records contain information about suggestions that were made, fears the patient expressed, and possibilities that were discussed, in addition to tests actually done and specialist visits actually made. The accumulating anecdotal evidence suggests that some information used by insurers to deny insurance comes from fairly informal conversations with physicians and informal notes. One woman was denied disability income insurance on the basis of her father's Huntington's disease, although the application had nowhere asked about family medical history or risk of genetic disease. She later learned that her doctor had written her father's diagnosis on the folder and the office had photocopied the folder notes as well as the inside records for the insurer.[26] Another woman was denied life insurance after she had questioned her obstetrician about the possibility of Huntington's disease in her mother. The physician had made a note of this conversation in her medical record, which was subsequently sent to an insurer.[27]

Most practicing physicians are probably not very knowledgeable about the underwriting practices of insurers. They are probably inclined to make their records as complete as possible, partly because the norms of good practice call for complete records, and partly out of a general concern with being able to defend themselves in potential malpractice suits. If they are wavering about whether to enter a notation about something a patient mentions—such as a concern about a family history of genetic disease—they are more likely to act on the side of inclusion for the above reasons, than to be influenced by thoughts of protecting their patients from future adverse underwriting decisions.

The Medical Information Bureau

In addition to answering questions about their health and sources of medical care and granting insurers access to their medical records, applicants for life and health insurance must usually sign an authorization for the insurer to seek information from the Medical Information Bureau (MIB). MIB is an insurance industry-run data bank, accessible to nearly 800 member companies in the United States and Canada. Insurers not only check the MIB database to find out whether an applicant has some impairment or disease not disclosed on the application; they also report to the MIB any information turned up in the course of underwriting that suggests an applicant has any risk factors relevant to underwriting.

Even applicants who have never applied for health insurance might have a record with the MIB if they have ever applied for life insurance, because most life insurance is medically underwritten. Member companies send information acquired in the course of underwriting to the MIB *daily*,[28] so that the data bank is extremely up-to-date. Thus, despite common parlance about the "competitive private market" in insurance, the consumer faces a monopolist seller in the sense that insurers can choose their customers, and virtually all insurers have access to the same information about a potential customer.

The MIB, in its public information brochure, assures "consumers and public representatives" that an insurer may not decline an application or charge more for coverage solely on the basis of the MIB's illness codes.[29] In theory, when an insurer receives information from the MIB that is not disclosed in the application or its own investigation, it is supposed to conduct its own research. In practice, there appears to be very little restriction on insurance companies' use of information obtained from the bureau in underwriting decisions. Moreover, although the MIB has procedures for individuals to correct information in their files, the procedures are cumbersome and it is often difficult for consumers to find out why they have been denied insurance in the first place.

Inspection Reports

Insurers sometimes request inspection reports from consumer reporting agencies. Investigators from an inspection agency interview friends, neighbors, and business associates, as well as the applicant, about the applicant's hobbies, lifestyle, financial situation, personal relationships, use of alcohol and drugs, driving record, and medical conditions. Un-

derwriters use these reports in part to obtain information about what
they call "unadmitted health histories." According to the major underwriting text, "In most cases, this information [unadmitted health his-
tories] comes from third parties via the inspection report. . . . "[30] If a
family were struggling with decisions about genetic testing because of
a family history of disease, it is very likely that they would discuss their
concerns with friends and possibly some neighbors who are also friends.
Thus, an insurance company might very well find out about a family
history of genetic disease via the inspection report.[31]

In sum, the industry's standard procedures of medical underwriting
entail extensive information gathering and information sharing, not
only among all companies, but also between its life and health insurance branches. Medical records from any medical source, as well as
health information from lay people, are widely available to, and used by,
insurers. Such sharing creates numerous avenues by which insurers will
inevitably acquire information about individuals' genetic make-up and
family history, *even if insurers do no testing of their own and ask no specific
questions about genetic disease.*

The Prevalence and Impact
of Medical Underwriting

In public discussions about underwriting and access to health insurance, insurers claim that underwriting is a minor phenomenon. They
use the term *underwriting* to mean examination of individuals for the
purpose of selecting risks and pricing policies. Because most health insurance is sold to large employee groups, and because (insurers claim),
large groups are not medically underwritten, very few people are affected by medical underwriting or put at risk of losing access to health
insurance on account of their medical histories. Thus, the 1991 report
of the ACLI-HIAA Task Force on Genetic Testing asserts:

> Most health insurance is not individually underwritten and so ge-
> netic testing would have no effect on the vast majority of health
> insurance consumers. About 85–90 percent of health insurance is
> currently purchased through group plans which accept all full-
> time employees and dependents without evidence of insurability.[32]

The industry thus maintains that only 10 to 15 percent of people with
health insurance are subject to underwriting, but this estimate is very
misleading. First, 19 percent of workers who have employer-based coverage work for firms of fewer than 10 employees, where individual underwriting virtually always obtains. Another 17 percent work for firms

with between 10 and 25 employees, where individual underwriting is extremely common.[33] Second, over the last decade or so there has been a trend toward using individual underwriting with even larger employee groups. A 1990 survey of insurers by the Colorado Division of Insurance found a substantial degree of individual medical underwriting in large groups: 11 percent of all commercial accident and health insurers and nonprofits require individual medical underwriting for *all groups*, regardless of size; 18 percent underwrite groups up to 99 people; 25 percent underwrite groups up to 74 people; 33 percent underwrite groups of up to 49 people; and 40 percent underwrite groups of up to 24 people.[34]

A third reason the industry estimate of the prevalence of underwriting is too low is that it ignores a major device for acquiring medical information about employees in large groups without obtaining it directly from the employees. Insurers often require a large-group employer to submit simple medical information about individual employees and their dependents. This information is obtained through what are known as "risk finder questions" or "gatekeeper questions" on the master application for a group. Typically, one question asks whether, to the best of the employer's knowledge, any employee or dependent had claims over a certain amount (say $2,500 or $3,500) during the previous year or two years. Other questions ask about more specific, but still quite general medical problems among employees and their dependents. This kind of *quasi-individual medical underwriting* is very common. The Colorado survey found that nearly three-fifths of insurers require a risk factor questionnaire for groups up to 49 people; nearly half require the questionnaire for groups of up to 99 people; and nearly one-third require it for all groups, regardless of size.[35]

Though we still do not know exactly how many people are affected by medical underwriting, the number must be vastly greater than the 10–15 percent the industry claims. Consider that in 1989 about 44 percent of the workforce was self-employed or employed in firms of under 100 employees.[36] Of workers who *have* employer-based health insurance, 36 percent work in firms of 25 or fewer employees, and 60 percent work in firms of 100 or fewer employees.[37]

When an individual or group is found to have high risks for disease, insurers might do several things besides offering a standard policy (or treating the person as a "standard risk," in insurance terminology). In the individual market, insurers can reject the applicant altogether as "uninsurable"; accept the applicant but charge a higher premium ("substandard rates"); accept the applicant but exclude coverage for a disease or organ or body system (called an "exclusion waiver"); or apply *both* an exclusion waiver and substandard rates. Exclusion waivers, it might be noted, are a major contributor to under-insurance, because they deny coverage for precisely those medical conditions a person has and for which he or she is likely to need treatment.

In the group market the options are similar, but they also include treating some members of the employee group differently from others. Thus, an insurer can reject a whole group; accept most of the group but exclude individuals who are deemed high-risk; charge a higher rate for the whole group, or alternatively, increase the rates only for the high-risk individuals in the group; limit the conditions or amounts covered either for the whole group or for certain members of the group; or *both* limit coverage and charge higher rates.[38] Perhaps most important, because all insurance policies are contracts, usually for one year, insurers can change the terms of any policy yearly as they acquire new information about policyholders' medical conditions.

It is not easy to know what insurers *actually* do when faced with high-risk applicants, because underwriting is part of a firm's competitive strategy and no firm is eager to disclose its practices. We can get some indication of the impact of medical underwriting on access to health insurance from two surveys of health insurer underwriting practices. A 1987 Office of Technology Assessment survey found that within the commercial individual insurance market, where medical underwriting currently obtains, around 8 percent of applicants are rejected outright for medical reasons. Commercial insurers apply exclusion waivers to another 13 percent, charge higher premiums to 5 percent, and use both exclusion waivers and higher premiums for 2 percent.[39] Taking these groups together, fully 28 percent of applicants do not meet the medical criteria to qualify as standard risks.

The Colorado survey described earlier asked insurers what actions they took and which action they take most frequently in the group market. Over half the insurers (54 percent) mentioned rejection of the group as the action most frequently taken when underwriting turns up adverse results. Fifteen percent said their most frequent action was to accept the group but exclude the high-risk individuals. Another 15 percent said their most frequent action was to limit coverage of high-risk individuals in the group.[40] Needless to say, each of these actions causes some people to be uninsured or underinsured.

Another way to estimate the impact of medical underwriting on access to health insurance is to determine what portion of the citizenry would be ineligible for standard risk insurance if they were subject to individual underwriting. The Citizen's Fund of Washington, D.C., used the underwriting manual of a large insurance company to identify medical conditions that would lead to denials, rating, or waivers, and then estimated the prevalence of those conditions in the general population from epidemiological surveys. Using this method, the study found that 81 million people under age 65 would not qualify for standard insurance if they had to submit to medical underwriting.[41]

In addition to traditional medical underwriting, there is a vast amount of retrospective underwriting after an insurance policy is in force. When an insured person or his or her medical provider submits a claim for payment, the insurer must make a decision whether to pay the claim. At this point, medical information enters again. The key vehicle here is the *preexisting condition clause*, a typical feature of most health insurance policies, even large group policies.

Preexisting condition clauses exclude payment for any condition the applicant had prior to the insurance contract. Preexisting conditions are generally defined in insurance policies as conditions which "manifested themselves," "existed," or "were treated" before the effective date of the policy. These words leave some leeway for interpretation, especially the "existed" criterion. Insurers have insisted on their right to refuse payment even for treatment of conditions which had not been diagnosed prior to the claim, and of which the applicant had no knowledge. Courts have often upheld insurers on this point.[42]

Preexisting condition clauses are far more potent than exclusion waivers and affect many more people. To write an exclusion waiver into a policy, insurers must detect some problem, from the applicant's medical records or the application, *in advance of issuing the policy*. The policy then specifically names the condition (or body part or system) as excluded. With the preexisting condition clause, insurers do not need any information about the applicant. The clause is like a wild card. It allows the insurer to refuse payment (tantamount to not insuring) for any condition the person had prior to the policy issue date, even when no information about the condition turned up in the medical underwriting process. Preexisting condition clauses thus have the same effect as exclusion waivers, without insurers having to do any underwriting at all, and unlike the exclusion waivers, they can be, and are, widely applied to group policies.

Yet another form of post-claims underwriting occurs when employers or insurers redesign the benefit package to exclude conditions for which a person has recently made claims. The most well-known instance of this strategy is the case of *McGann v. H & H Music Co.* After Mr. McGann filed his first claims for AIDS-related treatment, his employer switched from a commercial health insurance plan to a self-insured plan, and placed a $5,000 cap on payments for AIDS while leaving a $1 million maximum for all other treatment. The Court of Appeals for the Fifth Circuit ultimately upheld an employer's right to change its self-insured benefit plan in response to diseases or expenses incurred by a single employee.[43] Of course, an employer might do the same thing for any other disease. No doubt it would be harder for an employer to cap benefits for relatively common diseases that affect many employees and dependents, such as cancer or heart disease. But, like AIDS, genetic diseases tend to be less common and thus easier and more likely targets for employers looking for ways to cut the costs of their fringe benefits.

Commercial insurers effectively do the same thing when they push group members with expensive claims into reapplying for lower rates and submitting to medical underwriting. The insurer can then add an exclusion waiver, which is the equivalent of eliminating a disease from the benefit package for a self-insured group plan.

Restricting Insurers' Use of Genetic Information

The commercial life and health insurance industries have made it clear that insurers intend to use genetic information, at least insofar as it becomes available to consumers through the medical care system, and possibly by testing applicants themselves. Representatives of the industry have already announced they will resist any attempts by regulators or state legislatures to restrict their use of genetic information in underwriting.[44]

In response to public concern and pressure, the American Council of Life Insurance and the Health Insurance Association of America are promoting a program of confidentiality based on four "principles."[45] The program entails virtually no change from the current *modus operandi* of insurance companies, and would provide absolutely no more protection to insurance consumers than the status quo.[46] It addresses the problem of whether and under what circumstances an insurer may *redisclose* genetic information to a third party, but says nothing about whether and how an insurer may obtain such information or use it in making underwriting decisions. The trade associations take as a given that insurers will continue to collect genetic information, and will collect it and use it as in the same manner as they now collect and use all other medical information. Thus, the four principles of confidentiality all have to do with an insurer's redisclosure of individual information to other parties.

The most important principle is that (except in defined circumstances), a company may redisclose genetic information only "with the written consent or authorization" of the individual or his or her representative. The report suggests that "this consent could be obtained at the time an application is taken and would remain valid throughout the lifetime of the policy."[47] The consent would be "specific where possible, e.g., the MIB [Medical Information Bureau], and generic where otherwise necessary, eg. reinsurers, co-insurers, contractors, etc."[48] As we have seen, this is just the kind of written consent insurers already obtain on application forms; perhaps the committee contemplates adding specific mention of genetic information to the current standard waiver form. But even so, as we have also seen, the current "consent" is consent in name only. The applicant has no choice but to sign this waiver to release information because no company will consider an application without a signature of this waiver.

Many people concerned about the privacy issues as well as the insurance access issues raised by the Human Genome Project have proposed regulating insurers' use of genetic information in some fashion. Some have called for new state laws to prohibit insurers' use of genetic information in underwriting altogether.[49] Some have argued that state insurance commissioners should somehow regulate insurer practices in this sphere.[50] Others call for federal legislation, arguing that state jurisdiction might be too spotty or that insurance commissioners are unlikely to regulate these practices adequately.[51] The Task Force on Genetic Information and Insurance, a part of the Working Group on Ethical, Legal, and Social Implications of the Human Genome Project itself, called on insurers to "consider a moratorium on the use of genetic information in underwriting" until national health reform makes health care available to everyone regardless of present or future health status.[52]

Still others argue that we should distinguish between single-gene disorders, where a genetic defect definitively causes a disease, and genetic predispositions, and that we should prohibit only the first kind of genetic information in underwriting.[53] Another proposal would permit insurers to use genetic information in medical underwriting but use state "high-risk pools" to insure people who are medically uninsurable. These pools would be financed by some combination of individual premiums, state revenues, and payments by commercial insurers.[54]

None of these proposals, I believe, would begin to address the problems of health insurance access created by medical underwriting, and even the most stringent bans on insurer use of genetic information would probably be ineffective in curbing either the specific use of genetic information or the general problem of insurance denials and exclusion waivers. To start with the most permissive proposal, high-risk pools not only permit insurers to use genetic and other medical information to reject people, but *make it easier for insurers* to engage in risk-selection as a profit-seeking strategy by using state funds to subsidize care for the people whom insurers reject. In several states, even where insurers are assessed contributions to the high-risk pool, states allow the insurers to deduct these payments from their taxes. Self-insured employers cannot be taxed to support the pools, so that costly high-risk pools are another incentive for employers to self-insure, and pull out of risk-sharing arrangements with other employee groups. Moreover, high-risk pools have been in existence in 26 states for some years now, and they are barely making a dent in the uninsured population.[55]

Each of the other proposals entails some sort of ban on insurers' use of some or all genetic information. The problem with all of these proposals is that *genetic information is too deeply embedded in the structure of general medical underwriting to be effective regulated separately.* So long as the industry continues to use medical underwriting, it will be nearly impossible to prevent the use of genetic information. Genetic information about individuals is and will continue to be produced in the medical sector—in hospitals, laboratories, and doctors' offices. It will be recorded in physicians' records, in the form of written test results, family histories, informal talks, and physician referrals, recommendations, and advice. Even tests performed in commercial laboratories are likely to have some notation in physicians' records, and insurers' authorization to seek medical records are broad enough to encompass commercial laboratories anyway. Information about family genetic make-up will also be available to insurers through conversations with friends and neighbors in consumer credit agency inspection reports. So long as insurers are able to conduct general medical underwriting and compel applicants to release their medical records, genetic information will be available to them, even if some state or federal law prohibits them from using it as the basis of underwriting decisions.

If insurers *have* genetic information about individuals, legal prohibitions on its use in underwriting are unlikely to be easily enforced. Commercial insurers have demonstrated the intensity of their commitment to using this information in their published writing on the issue, in their fierce legislative lobbying on state and federal bills that curb underwriting prerogatives in any way, and in their actual behavior in the HIV testing controversy, where, when prevented from testing, they used the most statistically crude and discriminatory proxies to protect themselves from claims for AIDS. There is every reason to believe that insurers will use similarly crude family history information in lieu of genetic tests if they are prohibited from using genetic test results directly. Medical directors of large companies writing for the Committee on Genetic Testing of the ACLI have already acknowledged that insurers *do* use family history information as proxies, in the absence of good genetic tests.[56] Even if state or federal legislation also prohibited insurers from asking family history questions on application forms, insurers would still be likely to acquire this information from medical records.

Another way insurers might evade a prohibition on use of genetic information is by simply disguising their use of it. Insurers already make it difficult for applicants to find out why they are denied insurance by not volunteering this information in the first place. Typically, a consumer must ask the insurer in writing to release the reasons for rejection, and many companies will only release the information to a doctor. More importantly, insurers could simply find other reasons, besides genetic make-up, to find people uninsurable. One medical director of a large insurance company told the ELSI Task Force on Genetic Information and Insurance:

> If a woman has family history of breast cancer, I'll ignore the breast cancer. I won't rate her for the breast cancer, but I'll scrutinize her record extra carefully. I'll rate her for hypertension. I'll hope there is something else I can find in the record to rate her on. I'll tell her I rated her on hypertension. I won't tell her I rated her higher than someone else with the same hypertension.[57]

Medical underwriting decisions are highly discretionary and largely invisible. No legislative prohibition could reach the decision-making routines described by this underwriter, and consumers would be absolutely unable to police this kind of decision making.

Bans on the use of genetic information in underwriting would probably not reach post-claims underwriting. Even if insurers did not base an underwriting decision on genetic information, they could still deny claims at the payment stage for treatment of genetically based conditions by calling them preexisting conditions. Insurance law is based on state law, and there is as yet no settled doctrine on whether genetic or congenital conditions can be considered preexisting conditions by insurers for the purpose of nonpayment of claims. But judging from the kinds of insurance cases that get to court,[58] insurers probably will try to deny coverage for genetic conditions by using the preexisting condition clause. And again, policyholders are relatively powerless to police this kind of post-claims underwriting. Most do not have the knowledge, the financial resources, and sometimes the sheer physical energy to seek legal redress. Without an explicit statement in federal legislation making genetically based conditions not subject to preexisting condition clauses, insurers will often seek to deny payment for treatment of genetic diseases.

The *McGann* case discussed earlier illustrates how state-based prohibitions on genetic underwriting will be undermined. Under the Employee Retirement Income Security Act (ERISA), employers who self-insure are exempt from state insurance regulations (both statutory and regulatory). If commercial insurers are not allowed by state regulation or law to use genetic information, employers could evade this ban by self-insuring. Expensive but uncommon genetic diseases, such as Huntington's disease or Duchenne muscular dystrophy, might be limited or excluded from coverage.

As long as insurers continue to use general medical underwriting, insurers will continue to require applicants to authorize release of their medical records. This means the only way to attack the problem of insurer access to genetic information would be to control the flow of information from medical offices and facilities to insurers. Physicians usually photocopy the entire record or sections of the record in lieu of writing new reports to meet insurer requests. Any kind of legislative restriction on insurers' use of genetic information would therefore have to find a way to make physicians, hospitals, and other medical sources separate genetic information from other medical information. This would require major changes in the way physicians keep records. For example, not only specific test results but also conversations about family history, advice about genetic disease, and recommendations and referrals related to genetic disease would all have to be stored separately from the rest of the medical encounter. Clerical personnel would have to develop new record-keeping systems, and because they are the people who most often send records to insurers, they would have to be trained and supervised to protect genetic information. The room for slippage is enormous.

For all these reasons, preventing insurers from using genetic information in health insurance underwriting decisions is not so simple as creating a statutory or regulatory prohibition. It is doubtful whether it is possible to prevent the use of genetic information, or even some kinds of genetic information, without addressing the whole system of medical underwriting. If we are concerned about access to health insurance in the first place, then it makes sense to think about medical underwriting *per se*. After all, medical underwriting works to keep people who are sick or likely to be sick from obtaining private insurance at all or from obtaining coverage for those body parts, systems, and diseases for which they need medical care. Underwriting is a policy that makes perfect economic sense for the individual firm but is absolutely perverse to the individual and antithetical to the societal goal of universal access to health care. The Human Genome Project will have served a useful social purpose if it makes us reexamine the nation's commitment to our current private health insurance system.

Notes

1. Katherine Swartz, *The Medically Uninsured: A Special Focus on Workers*, Washington, DC, Urban Institute, 1989.

2. C. Nelson and K. Short, *Health Insurance Coverage 1986–88*. Bureau of the Census, U.S. Department of Commerce, Current Population Reports, Household Economic Studies, Series P-70, No. 17, March 1990, cited in Katherine Swartz and Timothy D. McBride, "Spells without Health Insurance: Distributions of Durations and Their Link to Point-in-Time Estimates of the Uninsured," *Inquiry*, vol. 27 (1990): 281–85.

3. U.S. Congress, Office of Technology Assessment, *Genetic Monitoring and Screening in the Workplace*, Washington, DC, 1990; Larry Gostin, "Genetic Discrimination: Employers and Insurers," *American Journal of Law and Medicine*, vol. 15, nos. 1–2, 1991: 109–44, esp. 115–19; American Council of Life Insurance, *The Potential Role of Genetic Testing in Risk Classification*, Report of the Genetic Testing Committee to the Medical Section of the American Council of Life Insurance, Hilton Head, South Carolina, June 10, 1989 [hereafter cited as "ACLI, *Potential Role*"].

4. *Report of the ACLI-HIAA Task Force on Genetic Testing*, Washington, DC, American Council of Life Insurers and Health Insurance Association of America, 1991, pp. 5–6 [hereafter cited as "ACLI-HIAA Task Force"]. See also Robert Pokorski, "Public Relations and Government Issues," in ACLI, *Potential Role*, pp. 8–17, esp. pp. 9, 18.

5. See "ACLI-HIAA Task Force," ibid.; Steven Brostoff, "CEOs: Defend Genetic Test Use in Underwriting," *National Underwriter—Life and Health Edition*, April 27, 1992, p. 27; Brian Cox, "Genetic Tests Become Next Underwriting Frontier," *National Underwriter—Life and Health*, July 27, 1992, pp. 3, 6; Jude Payne, Letter to the Editor, *National Underwriter—Life and Health*, September 27, 1992, pp. 41, 44.

6. For a comprehensive treatment of these arguments, and the analysis on which most subsequent writing about risk selection relies, see Herman T. Bailey, Theodore M. Hutchison, and Gregg R. Narber, "The Regulatory Challenge to Life Insurance Classification," *Drake Law Review* vol. 25, no. 4 (1976): 779–827.

7. Philip Stano, "Trifling with the Risk Classification System," *Journal of Insurance Regulation*, vol. 9, no. 4 (June, 1991): 542–74; quotation on p. 543.

8. American Academy of Actuaries, testimony, hearing on "The Rising Cost of Private Health Insurance: The Rating System," Committee on Energy and Commerce, Subcommittee on Commerce, Consumer Protection, and Competitiveness, U.S. House of Representatives, 102d Cong., 1st sess., April 30, 1991, pp. 1–2.

9. Robert I. Mehr, *Fundamentals of Insurance*, Homewood, IL: Richard D. Irwin, 1983, p. 439.

10. Robert J. Pokorski, "Public and Government Relations Issues," in ACLI, *Potential Role*, quotation on pp. 9–10.

11. Mark Battista, "Genetic Data: Impact on Underwriting," in ACLI, *Potential Role*, pp. 23–24. See also "ACLI-HIAA Task Force," p. 8, esp. n.4.

12. Battista, ibid., p. 26.

13. U.S. Congress, Office of Technology Assessment, *Medical Testing and Health Insurance*, Doc. No. OTA-H-384. Washington, DC: U.S. Government Printing Office, 1988, p. 64.

14. Benjamin Schatz, "The AIDS Insurance Crisis: Underwriting or Overreaching?" *Harvard Law Review*, vol. 100 (1987): 1782–1805, p. 1787.

15. Karen A. Clifford and Russell P. Iuculano, "AIDS and Insurance: The Rationale for AIDS-Related Testing," *Harvard Law Review*, vol. 100 (1987): 1806–25, p. 1810. For an extensive discussion of concepts of fairness in insurance, see Deborah A. Stone, "The Rhetoric of Insurance Law: The Debate Over AIDS Testing," *Law and Social Inquiry*, vol. 15, no. 2 (1990): 385–407; and Norm Daniels, "Insurability and the HIV Epidemic: Ethical Issues in Underwriting," *The Milbank Quarterly*, vol. 68, no. 4, 1990: 497–525.

16. Philip Stano, "Trifling with the Risk Classification System," p. 546.

17. Clifford and Iuculano, "AIDS and Insurance," p. 1808.

18. See "ACLI-HIAA Task Force," p. 6:

   Above all, it can not be emphasized enough that insurers are not using genetic tests in risk assessment, nor are there any plans to do so.

19. U.S. Congress, Office of Technology Assessment, *Medical Testing in Health Insurance*, p. 69; and table 2-12, p. 72 and figure 2-2, p. 73; see generally, Richard Baily, *Underwriting in Health and Life Insurance Companies* (Atlanta: Life Office Management Association, 1985).

20. Battista, "Genetic Data," p. 26. Emphasis added.

21. Pokorski, "Government and Public Relations Issues," p. 15 (emphasis added). See a similar point by Mark Battista: If genetic test results were incorporated into medical underwriting, " . . . [a]t least some applicants

whose family history or other medical data would previously have generated a declination would become insurable." Battista, "Genetic Data," p. 25.

22. Battista, in ACLI, *Potential Role*, p. 27.

23. This language is from a "typical form" reproduced in one of the textbooks used by the Health Insurance Association of America in its short courses for insurance education. Health Insurance Association of America, *Individual Health Insurance*, part A. Washington, DC, HIAA, 1991 ed., p. 135.

24. As part of a larger project, I am interviewing physicians and their staffs about their reporting practices with respect to insurers. Information here is gleaned from these interviews.

25. Gina Kolata, "New Insurance Practice: Dividing the Sick from the Well," *New York Times*, March 4, 1992, pp. A1 and A5.

26. Letter from Theresa Morelli, October 11, 1991, reprinted in U.S. House of Representatives, Committee on Government Operations, *Designing Genetic Information Policy: The Need for an Independent Policy Review of the Ethical, Legal, and Social Implications of the Human Genome Project*. 102d Cong., 2d sess. House Rept. 102-478. April 2, 1992, p. 16.

27. "Domestic and International Data Protection Issues," Hearings before the Subcommittee on Government Information, Justice and Agriculture of the Committee on Government Operations, U.S. House of Representatives, 102d cong., 1st sess., October 17, 1991, Testimony of Dr. Paul Billings, p. 247.

28. Bailey, *Underwriting*, p. 86; Charles A. Will, *Life Company Underwriting*, New York: Life Office Management Association, 1974, p. 50.

29. Medical Information Bureau, Inc., *A Consumer's Guide to the Medical Information Bureau*, Westwood, Mass. p. 7.

30. Bailey, *Underwriting*, p. 78.

31. While inspection reports are used less commonly in health insurance underwriting than in life, they are still used to a significant extent in individual and small-group insurance. See U.S. Congress, Office of Technology Assessment, *Medical Testing and Health Insurance*, p. 63. Moreover, the information from inspection reports would easily find its way to an underwriter of health insurance if the applicant had ever applied for life insurance, because any "reportable" information would have been entered into the bureau's files.

32. "ACLI-HIAA Task Force" p. 5.

33. Figures from the 1987 National Medical Expenditure Survey, cited in Health Insurance Association of America, *Health Care Financing for All Americans: Private Market Reform and Public Responsibility* (Washington, DC, 1991), p. 7, fig. 1.

34. Barbara Yondorff, *Health Insurance Availability and Affordability in Colorado: A report on underwriting and pricing practices*. Denver: Colorado Division of Insurance, 1990, p. 15, table 8.

35. Ibid., p. 15, table 9.

36. Citizens Fund, *Health Insurance at Risk* (Washington, DC, 1991) p. 22, table 4 (calculated from Current Population Survey, March 1990; figures are for 1989).

37. HIAA, *Health Care Financing*, p. 7; figures from 1987 National Medical Expenditures Survey.

38. In some states, insurers are required to accept or reject an entire group, and it is in these states that they are likely to reject a group with a few sick or high-risk members, because they cannot control the membership of their insured pool.

39. U.S. Congress, Office of Technology Assessment, *Medical Testing and Health Insurance*, p. 62.

40. Yondorff, *Health Insurance Availability*, p. 16.

41. Citizen's Fund, *Health Insurance at Risk*, p. 8. The study excluded people over 65 because they are eligible for Medicare with no medical underwriting.

42. *Dear v. Blue Cross of Louisiana*, 511 So. 2d. 73 (La. App. 1987) (insurer entitled to deny payment for a condition that predated the effective date of the policy, even though there had been no diagnosis or treatment but only symptoms); *Hanum v. General Life and Accident Ins. Co.*, 745 S.W. 2d 500 (Tex. App. 1988) (insurer may deny payment under preexisting condition clause for a condition which though not diagnosed prior to the policy, manifested itself in symptoms from which one learned in medicine could diagnose such a sickness or illness). See also Candace Goldstein, "Pre-existing Condition Medical Exclusion," *For the Defense* 30 (June 1988), pp. 2–7.

43. *McGann v. H & H Music Co.*, 946 F.2d 401 (5th Cir. 1991); cert denied, 113 S. Ct. 482 (1992) (upholding rights of employers, under ERISA, to make changes in benefit plans).

44. See note 5 above and accompanying text.

45. This strategy is outlined in American Council of Life Insurance, Subcommittee on Privacy Legislation to the Task Force on Genetic Testing, *Genetic Test Information and Insurance: Confidentiality Concerns and Recommendations*, American Council of Life Insurers, Washington, DC, 1992.

46. The Task Force said as much in its report (ibid., p. 7): "Although the Task Force enthusiastically endorses these principles, it must be emphasized that they are largely a reaffirmation of existing industry practices."

47. Ibid., p. 4.

48. Ibid.

49. See, e.g., Marvin R. Natowicz, Jane K. Alper, and Joseph A. Alper, "Genetic Discrimination and the Law," *American Journal of Human Genetics*, vol. 50, 1992: 465–75, p. 473. Paul Billings et al., "Discrimination as a Consequence of Genetic Testing," *American Journal of Human Genetics*,

vol. 50, 1992: 476–82, p. 481; Robert Lowe, "Genetic Testing and Insurance: Apocalypse Now?" *Drake Law Review*, vol. 40, no. 3, 1991: 507–32, p. 531.

50. Lowe, ibid.

51. Joseph Miller (comments), "Genetic Testing and Insurance Classification: National Action Can Prevent Discrimination Based on 'Luck of the Genetic Draw,'" *Dickinson Law Review*, vol. 93, no. 4, 1989: 729–57, pp. 75ff. See also, H.R. 2045, U.S. House of Representatives, 102d cong., 1st session (a bill to safeguard individual privacy of genetic information).

52. *Genetic Information and Health Insurance*, Report of the Task Force on Genetic Information and Insurance, NIH/DOE Working Group on Ethical, Legal, and Social Implications of Human Genome Research, National Institutes of Health NIH 93-3686, May 10, 1993.

53. Marne E. Brom, "Notes: "Insurers and Genetic Testing: Shopping for that Perfect Pair of Genes," *Drake Law Review*, vol. 40, no. 1 (1991): 121–48, pp. 145–46. Dennis S. Karjala, "A Legal Research Agenda for the Human Genome Initiative," *Jurimetrics Journal of Law, Science, and Technology*, vol. 32, no. 2, (Winter 1992): 121–222, p. 176.

54. Naomi Obinata, "Genetic Screening and Insurance: Too Valuable an Underwriting Tool to be Banned from the System," *Santa Clara Computer and High Technology Law Journal*, vol. 8 (May 1992): 145–76, pp. 161ff.

55. U.S. General Accounting Office, *Health Insurance: Risk Pools for the Medically Uninsurable*. Washington, DC, April 1988, Document No. GAO/HRD-88-66BR; U.S. General Accounting Office, *Access to Health Insurance: State Efforts to Assist Small Businesses*. Washington, DC, May 1992, Document No. GAO/HRD-92-90, esp. pp. 46–50.

56. See note 21 above and accompanying text.

57. Comments of a medical director at meeting of the Task Force on Insurance of the Ethical, Legal, and Social Issues Commission of the Human Genome Initiative, December 2, 1991, Bethesda, Maryland.

58. See *Goshorn v. Hospital Care Corporation*, 46 Ohio App. 3d. 47 (1989) (a preexisting condition in a hospital insurance policy did not apply to a congenital mitral valve condition that did not become manifest until after the effective date of the policy). The important thing to notice about this case is that the insurer *tried to deny payment* by labelling a congenital condition a preexisting condition. Insurers probably do this frequently, but few people fight in court.

Eight

Genetics and Employment
More Disability Discrimination

Adrienne Asch

In a book about the impact of the Human Genome Project on access to health care, there may be a moment's question about the place of an article on the effects of "the genetic revolution" (NIH/DOE, 1993, 1) on employment. However, as soon as it is recalled that 64 percent of Americans under age 65 who have health insurance coverage obtain that coverage through their connection to employment (Institute of Medicine, 1993), it should be clear that genetic information may affect employment status, and thereby access to health care as well. Accordingly, this chapter first discusses the more general topic of genetic information and employment before turning to the specific topic of genetic information and employer-provided health insurance. Before laying out the details, I state the positions that I shall argue.[1]

First, I believe that, fundamentally, how we deal with genetic knowledge—for good or ill—depends upon how we have historically and how we choose in the future to deal with disability, whatever its etiology. In saying this I do not deny that we must sometimes distinguish between genetic and nongenetic conditions; between single-gene and multifactorial ones; and between being affected with a condition and being someone who carries the gene for the condition. Notwithstanding these distinctions, I contend that we must craft our future policy to deal justly with all those who have disabling conditions, regardless of how those conditions came into existence.

Second, whether or not discrimination on the basis of genetic characteristics is interpreted to be part of such disability civil-rights legislation as the Americans with Disabilities Act, and whether or not the act is vigorously enforced, people who carry genes for disabilities or illnesses, and people who themselves are affected by those conditions, are likely to experience employment problems that the civil-rights laws are not designed to solve. Remedying these problems depends upon once and for all ending the link between having a job and getting acceptable health care. Until that link is severed, it is in an employer's self-interest—but not in the individual's or the nation's interest—to exclude people from the workforce. Thus, ending the link between one's job and one's medical coverage is a major step to ending the potential for excluding capable people from working, and simultaneously ameliorating the mental and physical problems that stem from prolonged, involuntary unemployment.

Third, even in the unlikely event that health reform removes access to health insurance from employment status, we must care about the consequences of genetic knowledge for the labor force potential of millions of our nation's people. To be denied the opportunity to work when one needs and wants to work is to deprive people of a substantial life activity with grave consequences for their own and for the nation's material and psychological well-being. Breaking this link gives people not only better health coverage; it also gives them a chance at better health.

Employment, Disability, and Genetics

In June 1994, the Bureau of Labor Statistics (BLS) reported that 6 percent of the nation was unemployed. When the bureau announces the nation's current unemployment rate, that rate is always far lower than the actual number of people who are not working but who would prefer to be doing so. To be counted as unemployed, an individual must be actively looking for work. Thus, all those who have stopped seeking jobs because they have been told that their education, skills, or their health disqualify them for the work available are not counted as among the officially unemployed.[2] In 1986, when Louis Harris and Associates conducted its first nationwide survey of people with disabilities, it reported that only one-third of respondents who were of working age were actually employed. Most of the 66 percent who were unemployed were not counted by the BLS as unemployed because they were not actively looking for work. Yet according to the same Harris survey, two-thirds of the 66 percent of the disabled who were unemployed would prefer to be working and believed that they were capable of working despite being classified as having a disability. The Louis Harris findings suggest that in the mid-1980s some eight million people with disabilities were chronically unemployed. Had these and other discouraged workers made it into the BLS data, then and now the unemployment rate would be substantially higher than 6 percent.

I do not intend here to evaluate the competing explanations for the staggering rates of nonparticipation in the labor force of the nation's disabled people. Undoubtedly, some of the twelve million had physical or cognitive disabilities so severe that they were genuinely unable to attempt work. However, then and now, unemployed disabled people point to such obstacles as lack of transportation, inaccessible workplaces, fear of loss of federally-provided medical care available under the Medicare program, and instances of employer rejection.

Americans with Disabilities Act

In supporting the 1990 Americans with Disabilities Act (ADA), a Democratic Congress and a Republican president acknowledged that people with disabilities were victimized by substantial, pervasive discrimination in all areas of life, including employment. Title I of the ADA bars employers from using an applicant's or employee's disability as a reason for denial of opportunity if the individual can, with or without reasonable accommodation, perform the essential functions of the job. Furthermore, employers may not deny to disabled employees any of the fringe benefits made available to the nondisabled. The ADA recognizes that myths and fears about people with disabilities have proven as limiting to full participation in social and working life as a physiological or cognitive limitation. Employers may no longer base their treatment of the disabled person on alleged discomfort of nondisabled co-workers and customers in the presence of someone with a disability; on undocumented claims that a disabled worker will threaten the health and safety of others; on unsubstantiated assertions that performing certain job tasks will endanger the health and safety of the disabled person; or on the conviction that disabled workers will perform less well and be absent more often than the nondisabled.

Congress was aware that employers might act on records of past health problems or on predictions about future ones. Accordingly, the ADA also forbids rejection or different treatment based on a record of a disability or on the knowledge that someone has a condition that is not now disabling but might be disabling at some time in the undetermined future. Thus, someone with a record of cancer in remission, or a previous psychiatric hospitalization, and someone with a progressive disease such as diabetes or multiple sclerosis, are all protected from denials of present opportunity based on past or future health problems.[3]

The foregoing comments apply to people with the full range of disabilities, regardless of their age of onset or their etiology. As we learn more about the role of genes in health and disease, ever-larger numbers of people who never before were perceived as disabled will discover that their genetic characteristics lead them to be viewed as disabled by others—notably employers and insurers. Their past, represented by medical records and family histories, and their future, revealed by tests detecting carrier status or predisposition to late-onset conditions, may be used against them to block attainment of their present goal of work.

In broad outline, genetic tests provide information about three types of individuals:

(1) people who are now asymptomatic but very probably will acquire disabilities from adult-onset conditions such as Huntington's disease, myotonic dystrophy, amyotrophic lateral sclerosis, and adult polycystic kidney disease;[4]

(2) people who, though currently asymptomatic, are predisposed—although not certain—to develop heart disease, diabetes, colon cancer, depression, or schizophrenia; and

(3) people who will never themselves have, but who carry genes for, such conditions as hemophilia, Duchenne muscular dystrophy, sickle cell anemia, cystic fibrosis, and Tay-Sachs disease, that they could pass on to their children.

In the employment context, the genetic information obtained and evaluated is collected in much the same way and used for the same purposes as all other medical information and should be viewed, therefore, merely as one type of medical information. Employers obtain all such data from applicants and workers at several times, and the ADA restricts them on when and how they may gather and use it. To forestall rejection of disabled applicants based on non-job-related medical information, the ADA prohibits any pre-offer medical history-taking, medical inquiry, or medical examination. However, it does permit employers to obtain medical information from prospective and current employees. After a conditional offer of employment, an employer may require all applicants to undergo medical examinations if all individuals in a particular job category are examined and if the medical records are stored in separate files and kept confidential. The employer may withdraw the offer if the individual is unable to perform the essential functions of the job. Employers also may conduct periodic examinations of all employees, but these examinations must be either limited to job-related medical conditions or voluntary.

Employers have legitimate, nondiscriminatory reasons for seeking medical information about prospective and current workers. Just as many jobs have educational prerequisites and skill requirements, so, too, many jobs require that people demonstrate physiologic, sensory, and perhaps neurologic abilities that are discerned most efficiently by a medical examination. In addition, as more and more evidence accumulates about the toxic effects of certain work environments, employers may wish to monitor the health of those continually exposed to known hazards (Natowicz and Alper, 1991).

Unfortunately, the Equal Employment Opportunity Commission (EEOC), which enforces the ADA, does not compel employers to limit their medical inquiries and examinations of conditional offerees to topics bearing only on the physical requirements of specific jobs (Equal Employment Opportunity Commission, 1991, 1630.14). For example, a woman applying for a middle-management job and a man seeking maintenance work may find that the exams they are given for the job are as broad and thorough as the ones they take at their private physician or HMO. Through the genetic testing that could become as routine as blood testing is now, the employer could learn that the currently healthy twenty-five-year-old M.B.A. or service worker could develop breast cancer or heart disease sometime in the next decade or two.

According to the ADA and its implementing regulations, such medical information must be kept confidential and maintained separate from other personnel records.[5] Although physicians are permitted to collect whatever information they think necessary at the post-offer stage, they are supposed to limit what they communicate to the personnel office to information bearing directly on current ability to perform specific tasks. The employer that decided against hiring the service worker or failed to promote the middle manager because of prognosis of severe disability many years in the future would have violated the law, but the mere fact that the employer is entitled to ferret out such information leads to apprehension about how the organization will use it.

As others have pointed out (Gostin, 1991), individuals whose offers are withdrawn after a medical examination have few avenues for getting sufficient information about the employment situation to successfully challenge the employer's change of mind. Because the post-offer medical examination takes place before the applicant is on the job, there is no way for the prospective employee to pin a sudden withdrawal of the offer to the examination results. Current workers who submit to periodic medical examinations as part of worksite-sponsored health promotion programs confront even more ambiguity in determining whether any subsequent employment decisions are due to this medical information. Is there a connection between the prognosis of breast cancer and the failure to get a high-prestige assignment, transfer, or promotion, or was someone else more qualified?

The antidiscrimination law in Minnesota affords far better protection to people with all types of diagnoses merely by insisting that all employment-conducted medical examinations be strictly related to ascertaining current ability to perform a specific job. In both the private and public sectors, job-related preplacement examinations have been developed and have been used successfully. Thus, one way to curtail the practice of excluding people from work based on non-job-related genetic and other medical information is to ensure that employers cannot collect it. The EEOC should adopt a similar regulation, which limits medical examinations and inquiries to medical conditions that directly affect job performance (Juengst, 1991; Rothstein, 1990). Otherwise, the enforcing agency is currently giving employers latitude to conduct medical fishing expeditions and leaving open the possibility for genetic and other disability discrimination that the ADA is designed to prevent.

If adverse treatment of people based on genetic characteristics were confined to people who currently have the disorder or who are presymptomatic, there might be no reason to discuss genetic discrimination separately from disability in general. However, people in the third category, unaffected carriers of genetic disorders, potentially could suffer discriminatory treatment from employers that learn of their carrier status from DNA tests taken as part of routine post-offer or post-employment medical examinations. Employers need not even perform the tests themselves; they need only require individuals to release their personal medical files to the company. Concern about discrimination stemming from employer or insurer knowledge of carrier status fuels much of the literature and research on genetic privacy (Nelkin and Tancredi, 1989; Andrews and Jaeger, 1991) and the call for specific legislation to prohibit "genetic discrimination" (Billings et al., 1992).

People who carry genes for cystic fibrosis, sickle cell anemia, or hemophilia will never develop these particular impairments but may transmit them to their children. If post-offer and post-employment medical inquiries come to include DNA testing, employers will have access to even more non-job-related information about their workers and their workers' families. As students of disability tell us, employers and the public at large frequently discriminate against carriers of genetic conditions in the same way that they discriminate against the people who actually manifest them (Goffman, 1963). One common myth is to equate carrier status itself with actual disability or incapacity to meet some standard of functioning. "Discrimination against an unaffected carrier is particularly pernicious because the condition is irrelevant to the person's current or future health status or abilities. The discrimination is based on the mythology that a heterozygote has the disease or will develop it" (Gostin, 1991, p. 118).

Employers who exclude carriers of genetic conditions from their workforce, or who otherwise treat them in ways that distinguish them from those who are not known to carry genetic disabilities, are acting on medical information that is not job-related. They are either erroneously "regarding" the carriers as people with impairments; treating them as having a record of an impairment; or acting on some concerns about future risk—either the erroneous view that they will become disabled in the future and unable to perform, or the fear that they will draw heavily upon the employer-financed medical benefits.

Some of those particularly concerned about what they describe as "genetic discrimination" contend that it is distinct from and should be dealt with apart from legislation and policy intended to curtail disability discrimination (Billings et al., 1992; Billings et al., 1992a). Among several of their illustrations of genetic discrimination in employment, they describe the rejection of a prospective government worker who was identified as a carrier of the gene for Gaucher's disease, for which he was currently asymptomatic. Whether the rejection stemmed from concerns about future incapacity to perform tasks or fears about future extensive use of employer-provided benefits, the rejection was based on a perception of the problems of current or future disability. The etiology is immaterial to the employer's rejection. At the time this incident was reported, the Equal Employment Opportunity Commission did not interpret rejection based upon genetic predisposition as instances of disability discrimination covered by the Americans with Disabilities Act. Fortunately, in a March 1995 addition to its Compliance Manual, EEOC revised its prior interpretation concerning genetic predisposition to offer protection under the act, explaining that such individuals are "regarded" as having a disability.

The Genetic/Nongenetic Distinction

The expansion of genetic knowledge only strengthens my conviction that it is conceptually misguided, morally objectionable, and politically counterproductive to treat discrimination based on genetics with new legislation that distinguishes it from general disability discrimination. "As a practical matter it will become increasingly difficult to deal with genetic information as special and separate from other forms of health-related information because diseases are increasingly understood as having both genetic and environmental components" (NIH/DOE, 1992, 3).

At the moment that research links genes to diabetes, hypertension, arthritis, and other common disorders, virtually everyone will discover that he or she is "at risk" for some condition that can be regarded as a disability. Each one of us will be compelled to face the fact that we carry genes for conditions that will someday limit us or may limit our children. Much of the dismay about genetic information being used by employers is felt by those who have never questioned their own fitness, wellness, and employability when they realize that they may suddenly be regarded as unwell, unfit, and unemployable. In essence, they will be stigmatized and discriminated against just as people with other, already-detectable conditions have been excluded and discriminated against for centuries. They, too, will be victimized by many of the same demeaning stereotypes and excluded from the working world.

The hue and cry about genetic discrimination is a "them"–"us" phenomenon. Presymptomatic individuals are not now disabled, even if they may be sometime in the future. Carriers of x-linked or recessive conditions are not and will not be affected, even if their offspring could be affected. As genetic research has already revealed, however, carriers are everyone, ordinary people, the people in power. They are not the powerless, stigmatized, excluded disabled people who have been viewed as "them" or "the other" throughout history (Asch, 1989; Goffman, 1963; Miringoff, 1991). It may have been understandable to exclude, classify, or treat differently people with "real" disabilities; they really were different. To be singled out for harsh treatment based on being a carrier of a genetic condition is to become the different and stigmatized and to move from the "us" to the "them."

On the other hand, recognizing that genetic discrimination is just another form of disability discrimination is to bring home to everyone that there truly is no more "them" and "us." We all have characteristics that someone can consider frailties or problems that can be used by employers, insurers, or other institutions as a basis for discrimination. We understandably rebel against those who would impose needless restrictions upon our opportunities. Genetic discrimination, then, should be acknowledged as simply discrimination based on disability—disability that is manifest now; that will be manifest in the future; or that may be manifest in someone's future children.

In 1995 the EEOC issued an opinion that individuals who are discriminated against in employment because of genetic predisposition to disease are being regarded as having a disability and thus are covered under the third prong of the definition of disability under the ADA. While this is a positive development, it does not afford coverage to individuals who are unaffected carriers of recessive and x-linked disorders who also may be said to be regarded as having a disability.

Employment, Genetics, and the
Health Insurance Problem

As I have already mentioned, another rationale behind the denial of employment to people with disabilities has been the employer belief that disabled workers would draw disproportionately upon an employer's health and long-term disability insurance. Those who are wary of the misuse of genetic information in the employment context are understandably opposed to the exclusion of capable workers because employers learn that they, or their children, have conditions that will necessitate extensive and expensive medical care. Because employers now provide the health coverage for nearly two-thirds of those people who have health insurance of any kind (Institute of Medicine, 1993), they have a considerable economic investment in their workers' health and in the health of any dependents that they also cover. Employer concern about future risk, then, may be as much a concern about future risk of expensive pay-outs in health benefits as it is a concern about risk of future incapacity to meet job demands.

Employers trying to maximize their economic self-interest could use medical information about presymptomatic status, genetic predisposition to disease, genetically caused sensitivity to workplace carcinogens, or carrier status, to deny people work and to lay off or discharge current workers whose medical problems they discover. Even if employer examinations were revamped in the ways I have proposed, they could still learn about their workers' health and the health of their workers' families by reviewing health insurance claims—an increasingly common practice as more employers become self-insured.

The ADA does not indicate how workers' privacy is protected if they submit requests for reimbursement for medical services to the employer benefits office. Although the ADA insists that employee health records be maintained in a way to preserve confidentiality, benefit claims are not medical records. Moreover, it is too much to hope that someone who reviews the claim form about a genetic test for a rare disorder or about a stay in a psychiatric hospital will not comment upon that fact to someone in the organization. By word of mouth, without any traceable written record, the information can get to those in charge of hiring, firing, and promoting the employee.

The ADA, as interpreted by the EEOC's regulations, offers some protection to people with genetic and other medical conditions likely to incur substantial health care costs. The EEOC construes the law to prohibit an employer from making a decision about hiring, retention, or advancement based on the current or future costs of the employee's medical care or that of the employee's covered dependents. In its June 1993 memorandum on the subject of employer health insurance and the ADA, the EEOC stated that "decisions about the employment of an individual with a disability cannot be motivated by concerns about the impact of the individual's disability on the employer's health insurance plan" (Equal Employment Opportunity Commission, 1993). For example, if an applicant or employee could establish that an adverse decision was made following the revelation that the individual or a covered dependent was diagnosed with an expensive condition, be it a nongenetic cancer or a genetic one such as retinoblastoma, the individual could probably sustain a complaint filed under the law.

My reading of the law and its interpretive regulations leads me to wonder how the issues of "direct threat" to self (justifying exclusion from the workplace) and those of "future risk" (not justifying exclusion) will be harmonized. This matter could be especially significant for genetic-related conditions detected by monitoring the effects of exposure to workplace toxins. In other words, if it were possible to accurately determine that an individual was virtually certain to become severely disabled by prolonged exposure to carcinogens that were indispensable to the job, and that the threat of substantial harm could not be ameliorated by any reasonable accommodation, would an employer be justified in rejecting someone from undertaking the work? If the employee could continue to perform the job notwithstanding the impairment, denying the worker the employment opportunity based on legitimate concerns about the welfare of the worker or because the impairment would eventually (or soon) cost the employer money in lost productivity or increased health care costs would appear not to be a defense.

The EEOC interprets the ADA as permitting employers to exclude individuals from jobs which pose a direct threat of substantial harm to themselves or third parties. This interpretation differs from that made by some state civil rights agencies that have enforced disability antidiscrimination statutes for many years, and it also could be perceived as at variance with the Supreme Court's handling of fetal protection policies in its 1991 *United Auto Workers v. Johnson Controls, Inc.* case. I wonder whether the oft-stated concern for the health and safety of the individual with a genetic predisposition to workplace-caused impairment is, in many instances, actually a concern for the employer's pocketbook. Ideally, there will be sufficient work opportunities for someone to get out of work that is likely to harm his or her health, but in the absence of such opportunities, we should oppose the paternalism that will deprive people of their means of financial survival in the name of protecting their physical well-being.

To the extent that health insurance costs could be used by employers to exclude workers with disabilities and their dependents, the dependents may fare better than the workers themselves under the ADA and its interpretation. The ADA explicitly prohibits an employer from basing any employment decisions about individuals on their known relationships with people who have disabilities. Consequently, if an employed woman's husband has multiple sclerosis, or if the same woman's child has inherited hemophilia which she passed on to him, the employer cannot fire her or fail to advance her because the employer is incurring expenses resulting from the health of her dependents. Here, again, the same problems and protections needed by anyone who is financially responsible for someone with a disability are what should be considered, not whether the disability of the dependent is genetically transmitted by the employee.

The employer-provided health insurance problem goes beyond the adverse decisions an employer may make about the employment of a particular individual and actually must be understood as bearing upon the decisions they make about the scope of the health benefits they choose to provide to any of their workers. If employers wish to avoid incurring high-cost health care on behalf of workers and their families, they need only drop dependent coverage entirely (as many already have done) or scale down the types of medical conditions they will cover for their work force. Section 501(c) of the ADA permits employers to retain and devise health benefit plans that make certain types of distinctions in what they will cover. Employer-sponsored plans may, for example, exclude classes of disabilities such as mental disabilities or substance abuse treatments from their coverage altogether, or may set radically different lifetime benefits for coverage of mental versus physical disability. They may also exclude reimbursement for whole classes of services (such as blood transfusions or genetic testing) without violating the act. The EEOC does not view the creation of a benefit plan as discriminatory if its decisions can be justified on valid risk classification and underwriting principles, or if the employer can show that it can financially sustain its plan only by excluding certain classes of disorders.

Job-seekers already factor in an employer's benefit plan when selecting among alternative places to work. Employers can evade high-cost benefits and evade discrimination complaints simply by making it known that they do not cover many conditions and procedures. If such actions become widespread, the man who knows that he, his wife, or his child has an expensive, uncovered set of medical needs will effectively be precluded from working.

The employer that uses new genetic knowledge in constructing a benefit plan and determines legal methods of excluding an increasing variety of medical procedures and disorders from coverage merely exacerbates an existing problem faced by significant numbers of working people. These people cannot change their current jobs without losing their health insurance because they, or someone in their family, has a preexisting condition that a new employer's plan will exclude. The May 1993 report of the NIH/DOE Joint Task Force on the effects of genetic research on health insurance indicates that an estimated three in ten employees believe that they are compelled to stay in their current jobs simply to prevent the loss of necessary health insurance for themselves or their families (NIH/DOE, 1993, p. 19).

Ultimately, no tinkering with the ADA and its regulations or any new civil rights legislation protecting the carriers of genetic conditions can simultaneously promote employment for those with medical problems and promote the economic well-being of employers. For however long employers continue to finance health care for their workers, some employers will continue to find methods of excluding all but the people whose current or future health problems escape detection. Larry Gostin captures the coming catch-22 when he says: "The course currently charted by the Human Genome Initiative is filled with the promise of unimagined medical advancement for humankind. The potential harm to human beings by rendering them virtually unemployable or uninsurable may be equally real" (Gostin, 1991, p. 142).

Workers, labor unions, and employers must insist that financing health care should no longer be part of the employer-employee relationship. It is in everyone's interest to make employment decisions exclusively on whether people are qualified for and want to participate in the work at a particular organization. Everyone who cares about promoting employment and promoting the growth of the nation's economy should unite to demand that the financing of health care be forever removed from the connection to employment. Only some system of national health care reform that guarantees comprehensive services to all persons, regardless of their employment status or their medical need, will free employers to decide who is best suited for the work available, and will afford to job-seekers the opportunity to select work based on its likelihood of fulfilling their financial, psychological, and social needs. Workers should have the freedom to look for work based on the character of the work and the people involved, and not on the health coverage the work provides. Employers should strive for a workforce committed to the job to be performed. It is in everyone's interest to make work more productive for the individual, the employer, and the society. One substantial step is severing health care access from employment status.

Conclusion

These comments bring me to the message with which I wish to conclude this chapter: The principal focus of this chapter is on the consequences of genetic knowledge for employment and on employer-provided health care. Yet we must commit ourselves to more than affording medical services to our citizens. We must be concerned to ameliorate the pervasive social and health problems directly or indirectly attributable to chronic, involuntary unemployment. In addition to the extremes of violence, substance abuse, and mental illness that create the need for an ever-larger health and social service system, unemployment brings with it less serious but tangible problems for individuals and families: loss of self-esteem and social recognition, a sense of alienation from community, and a lack of purpose in life (Chestang, 1982; Perlman, 1982). The millions of people with disabilities who are currently out of work but not counted as unemployed suffer the social and psychological problems of this involuntary unemployment and undoubtedly add to the nation's health costs because of these psychological and social problems.

Health care reform along the lines proposed by the NIH/DOE Task Force would substantially improve access to health services for everyone. Such reform, along with the ADA, should remove the incentives of employers to reject individuals with current disabilities or with genetic indications of future disability. Keeping employed those who have long been in the work force, and reaching out to the millions who have been out of the labor market, would go a long way toward ameliorating the nation's health costs and to giving people a chance at better health.

Notes

1. My citations to Mark Rothstein cannot adequately indicate his intellectual contribution to this subject area in general and to this article in particular. His comprehensive knowledge of this topic infuses this article throughout,

and his thorough presentation in the article "Genetic Discrimination in Employment and the Americans with Disabilities Act" (1992) has helped me immeasurably to structure my own thinking.

2. There are, of course, other reasons why people who might prefer to work are no longer looking for jobs: no jobs requiring their skills exist in their geographic area and they are constrained to relocate; or they would not earn enough to offset expenses they would incur in hiring others to help with family and domestic responsibilities that they now discharge themselves.

3. For useful analyses of the requirements of the ADA, see, for example, West, 1991, and Asch and Watson, 1992.

4. Although both Huntington's chorea and some forms of familial breast cancer are single-gene disorders, they do not appear to be equally determinative of actually acquiring the condition. The work on breast cancer is much more recent than that on HD; it appears that 85 percent of those who possess the breast cancer gene on chromosome 17 will develop breast cancer before menopause. (McNeil-Leher News Hour, July 30, 1993).

5. See Andrews and Jaeger, 1991, for a comprehensive discussion of confidentiality of genetic information in the workplace that concludes with some proposals to strengthen it.

References

Andrews, L. B., and Jaeger, A. S. 1991. "Confidentiality of Genetic Information in the Workplace." American Journal of Law and Medicine, (1–2), 75–108.

Asch, A. 1989. "Reproductive Technology and Disability." In S. Cohen and N. Taub, eds., Reproductive Laws for the 1990s (Clifton, NJ: Humana Press), 69–125.

Asch, A. and Watson, S. 1992. "Federal Legislation Affecting Disability Management Practices." In S. H. Akabas, L. B. Gates, and D. Galvin, eds., Disability Management (Washington, DC: ANACON Publishers), 22–64.

Billings, P. R., Kohn, M. A., deCuevas, M., Beckwith, J., Alper, J. S., and Natowicz, M. R. 1992. "Discrimination as a Consequence of Genetic Testing." American Journal of Human Genetics, vol. 50, 476–82.

Billings, P. R., Alper, J. S., Beckwith, J., Barash, C. I., and Natowicz, M. R. 1992a. "Letter to the Editor: Reply to Hook and Lowden: The Definition and Implications of Genetic Discrimination." American Journal of Human Genetics, vol. 51, 903–905.

Chestang, L. W. 1982. "Work, Personal Change, and Human Development." In Sheila H. Akabas and Paul A. Kurzman, eds., Work, Workers, and Work Organizations: A View from Social Work. (Englewood Cliffs, NJ: Prentice-Hall), 61–89.

Equal Employment Opportunity Commission, 1991. Compliance Manual, vol.

2. EEOC order 915.002, Definition of the Term "Disability," at 902-45, March 15, 1995. Reprinted in *Daily Labor Reporter*, March 16, 1995, at E1, E23.

Equal Employment Opportunity Commission. 1993. "Text: Interim Guidance on Application of ADA to Health Insurance." 6/9/93 (No. 109). (Washington, DC: Bureau of National Affairs, 20037), E-1-E5.

Goffman, E. 1963. *Stigma: Notes on the Management of Spoiled Identity.* (Englewood Cliffs, NJ: Prentice-Hall).

Gostin, L. 1991. "Genetic Discrimination: The Use of Genetically Based Diagnostic and Prognostic Tests by Employers and Insurers." American Journal of Law and Medicine, vol. 17, (1-2), 109-44.

Louis Harris and Associates. 1986. ICD Survey of Disabled Americans: Bringing Disabled Americans into the Mainstream. (New York: Louis Harris and Associates); Study Number: 854009.

Institute of Medicine, National Academy of Sciences. 1993. Employment and Health Benefits (Washington, DC: National Academy Press), 28.

Juengst, E. T. 1991. "Priorities in Professional Ethics and Social Policy for Human Genetics." JAMA, vol. 266, 1835.

Miringoff, M. L. 1991. *The Social Costs of Genetic Welfare.* (New Brunswick, NJ: Rutgers University Press).

National Institutes of Health–Department of Energy Working Group on the Ethical, Legal, and Social Implications of Human Genome Research. "Genetic Information and Health Insurance: Report of the Task Force on Genetic Information and Insurance." May 10, 1993 (pre-publication copy).

Natowicz, M. R. and Alper, J. S. 1991. "Genetic Screening: Triumphs, Problems, and Controversies." Journal of Public Health Policy, vol. 12, no. 4.

Perlman, H. H. 1982. "The Client As Worker: A Look at an Overlooked Role." In Sheila H. Akabas and Paul A. Kurzman, eds., *Work, Workers, and Work Organizations: A View from Social Work.* (Englewood Cliffs, NJ: Prentice-Hall), 90-116.

Rothstein, M. A. 1990. "Recommendations for Regulations to Implement the Americans with Disabilities Act." Letter submitted to the Equal Employment Opportunity Commission, November 20 (unpublished), 1-6.

Rothstein, M. A. 1992. "Genetic Discrimination in Employment and the Americans with Disabilities Act." Houston Law Review, vol. 29, 1, 23-84.

U.S. Department of Labor, Bureau of Labor Statistics. 1992. "The Unemployed: Who They Are and How They Are Counted." January.

West, J., ed. 1991. The Americans with Disabilities Act: From Policy to Practice. (New York: Milbank Memorial Fund).

Nine

The Human Genome Project and the Distribution of Scarce Medical Resources

Norman Daniels

Three Questions about Resource Distribution

The human genome project has important implications for the distribution of scarce medical resources, whether they are naturally scarce, like bodily organs, or "socially" scarce, because of reasonable limits on what can be spent on health care. Just what these implications are will depend, I shall argue, on facts about the design of our health care system, including the reforms we make in the near future. I shall also suggest that the genome project does not raise completely novel issues of resource allocation. It will, however, make it more urgent that we address some issues we already face. I shall not discuss the most obvious resource implication of the genome mapping project, its "opportunity cost." By investing in the genome project, we give up the opportunity to produce other health benefits that would result from alternative research and development projects. The same point can be raised about the technologies that arise from the genome project itself. Each of these raises the question, Are we better off developing this technology or using our resources in some other way? I ignore the issue of opportunity costs since there is nothing distinctive about the way in which it arises for the genome project (Daniels, 1988).

173

I shall discuss in turn three implications of the genome project for the distribution of resources. The first two implications derive from the fact that the genome project will enhance our ability to predict an individual's health risks, not only with regard to genetic diseases, but also for other diseases whose genotypic contribution we have been unaware of or could only estimate from family history. The third implication derives from the fact that the genome project may increase our ability to enhance human capabilities rather than merely lead to treatments for disease. I will concentrate on a key moral question that bears on each of these resource implications.

First, consider the allocation of some naturally scarce resources, like bodily organs. If we can better predict outcomes of transplant procedures, for example by knowing who is likely to survive without other health problems later in life, then we sharpen a long-standing debate about the appropriate criteria for patient selection for transplant procedures: *What weight should we give to assuring "best outcomes" rather than giving people "equal chances at an important benefit"?*

Second, our enhanced ability to screen for health risks can reduce access to medical services of those at risk if standard underwriting practices exclude them from health insurance coverage. These practices mean that the people most likely to need certain services will find it hardest to get them, while those at lowest risk will gain economic advantage. Alternatively, in a system in which there was universal access to insurance, screening could serve to increase access to medical services. The genome project thus makes it more urgent that we address the moral question underlying standard underwriting practices: *What are our moral obligations to share these risks despite improved information about them?*

Third, by giving us a better understanding of the genetic factors that underlie human variation in capabilities, for example, by allowing us to look at the microstructure underlying the "normal distribution" of height, the genome project may increase demand to enhance certain capabilities where we can. It may lead us to classify certain genes as "undesirable" and produce pressures for us to modify their effects. This will pose a special challenge to the traditional distinction between treatment and enhancement, a distinction which traditionally limits our obligations to provide people with medical services. *Can we defend the distinction between medical therapies that treat and those that enhance in the face of new genetic information that allows us to pinpoint the genetic contributors to traits we want to alter?* This question takes us deep into political philosophy, for we are really asking, Which inequalities between people give rise to claims on others and which are matters of individual responsibility?

Should We Favor Best Outcomes or Equal Chances?

In some contexts of significant scarcity, whether natural or social, providing a benefit to some means others will not receive it. In some triage situations, for example, we may have to choose whether or not to award an ICU bed to the patient with the best prospects of survival when we know that not getting the ICU bed reduces both patients' chances significantly. In our prevailing patient selection protocols for organ transplantation, the likelihood of a "better outcome" earns "points" toward selection. Imagine, then, that genetic screening gives us new information reliable to estimating the outcome, especially long-term, of giving one patient an organ rather than another. What weight should we give this information in the distribution of scarce, lifesaving resources?

Two plausible goals seem to conflict when we think about the design of eligibility and selection criteria for organ transplantation. One goal is to use the scarce resource to produce a good outcome. The other is to give a fair chance to all people who might benefit from the transplanted organ. Few people seem to be attracted to pursuit of either goal in the extreme, as Brock (1988:94) notes. We would be reluctant to break a tie in choosing between two patients because one has more relatives who would be happy if she survived or because one is likely to live 40 years and the other only 37. These differences, we probably think, do not justify reducing the chances of one relative to the other of receiving the transplant. Similarly, we are unlikely to insist on equal chances—a lottery—to decide between selecting a healthy young woman who can be restored to full functioning for a normal lifespan and selecting a 75-year-old man with little likelihood of surviving the operation and who is likely to die of an unrelated condition in two years anyway. But these examples only raise the general question: When and on what grounds can a fair procedure allow departures from assuring people equal chances at receiving the benefit a transplant will give them? This is a complex issue. Not only are our moral intuitions complex and varied, but the underlying theory about what constitutes fairness is also complex and controversial.

We cannot hide from this issue by appealing to "medical criteria" and thinking that they can solve the problem of selection in a value-neutral manner (Brock, 1988:88–89). To the extent that such factors as organ size, blood type, tissue typing, and donor-recipient cross-matching play a role in selection, they import judgments about when it is permissible to reduce equal chances at some benefit in favor of making sure that some threshhold benefit is achieved. To the extent that factors that go beyond immediate success—longevity and quality of life—also parade as "medical" criteria, even more controversial reductions in equal chances are involved.

The question, When are departures from equal chances fair? needs some motivation. Why start with equal chances at all? Suppose you and I both need a transplant. For you, it is only likely to yield a two-year extension of life; for me, it might yield twenty. You might say: "For me, the two years is everything. From the perspective of what is important to me, it is just as important as your living at all—for however long." Or change the example: the transplant has a 40 percent chance of immediate success for you and an 85 percent chance for me. You might still say, "I know I have a smaller chance at success, but why should I be given *no* chance, which is what I will have if you get the transplant." You might think that it is not just unfortunate or unlucky that your longevity or success is less than mine, but that it is unfair for the selection criteria to reduce to nothing your chances at survival by awarding the organ to me.

In its extreme form, this argument pulls us toward accepting nothing as a reason for reducing chances below equality. Consider the case of a recent triple transplant involving a second effort at a heart transplant. Suppose the three organs might have been used to save three other lives. The recipient might have argued as follows: "The triple transplant can save me or save the three of them. My chances at having my life saved should not be reduced below an equal chance to save one of theirs merely because an additional two lives can be saved if we save one of theirs?" I suspect that few of us accept this argument. On the other hand, we probably do feel the pull of this one: you have no siblings and I have one that cares about me deeply. You might well object that your chances of receiving the organ should not be made less than mine merely because of that difference in the goodness of the outcome if I receive the organ rather than you.

Two (non-exclusive) philosophical "methods" have been used to explore this issue. In a brilliant discussion of doctors and the allocation of scarce resources, Francis Kamm (1987) has tried to uncover the structure of our "ordinary morality" intuitions about hypothetical cases that strongly resemble the problem of selecting patients for transplants. For example, she examines cases in which we can choose to redirect a threat (a runaway trolley) or to direct a benefit (e.g., an organ or a medicine) to different groups of people. Her cases confirm that we would not, for example, break ties between people whose lives are at stake merely because of the chance to gain relatively minor additional goods, like curing a third person's sore throat. (The goods have to be "contestants.") We do choose, in these cases, to foresake equal chances when the tiebreaker consists of certain kinds of goods: for example, goods that people are not expected, or obliged, to sacrifice even to save the life of another, such as the loss of an arm. The gain of an extra twenty years of life might seem to fit this description, since we do not oblige people to sacrifice twenty years of their lives to save another, but our intuitions are actually more complex than this. Thus I would not be willing to break a tie between individuals I might save because, when I save one, he loses an arm, but when I save the other, he will be fully functional. This seems to be true even though I am willing to redirect a threat or direct a benefit that will save one life plus *another's* arm rather than merely save one life.

By exploring related cases, hoping to tease apart what the relevant differences are between them and what does the work in our intuitions, we can hope to uncover the structure of our ordinary moral views on the subject. More than that, by better understanding that structure, we might be able to see what really carries justificatory force. In that way, we might hope to be able to resolve cases in which people's intuitions conflict or are not clear. What Kamm shows us is that our ordinary moral intuitions combine both "objective" and "subjective" viewpoints. To some extent, we are willing to give up assuring individuals equal chances at some good because we are willing to some extent to weigh goods on an objective scale: we may count saving significantly more life years as a greater good than saving fewer life years. Nevertheless, we still respect the subjective view, paying some attention to the fact that an objectively smaller benefit denied to one individual will subjectively be viewed as a great loss by that individual, especially where life is concerned. We are not, then, indifferent to whose life is saved.

There is another approach philosophers have taken to the problem of fairness and departures from equal chances—an approach that is more theoretical, though it appeals to moral intuitions at other levels. Consider the following objection to someone who says that only a lottery (assuring equal chances) should be allowed to decide between himself and someone who faces a greater probability of success or who can expect more quality life years saved: "There is no need to run a lottery now. The fact that *you* and not the other has lower expectations of success is itself the result of a *natural lottery*. It is just random chance that it is you and not the other who has less likelihood of a good outcome. That natural lottery already gave you equal chances at being the one with the qualification for selection. There is no reason to run another lottery now merely because we know the outcome of the previous one." (I used this argument in the Battelle Institute project several years ago, and others have made similar points; cf. Brock, 1989, Kamm, 1987, 1989.) The issue here is whether the person who insists on the second lottery is really a sore loser in a fair competition (like the child who says "let's make it three out of four" after losing two out of three), or whether there is no fair competition that relies on such a natural lottery.

We might defend the claim that we should not have two lotteries in the following way. We should decide *ex ante* what will count as acceptable departures from equal chances. If it is reasonable to pick criteria that aim, within limits, at securing good results from transplants—because, *ex ante*, we would be better off living under a system that selected in that way—then those criteria constitute a fair procedure. Thus we might reason as follows in light of my earlier remark that a just health care system is one that protects fair equality of opportunity over the lifespan. Everyone, *ex ante*, has an improved chance of functioning normally over a normal lifespan if transplant selection criteria give some weight to outcomes that yield significantly more quality life years saved than outcomes that do not. If reasonable people, who do not know how they stand in the natural lottery (e.g., they do not know whether they need organs) could agree that such a system better uses resources to protect opportunity than an alternative system, say one with two lotteries, then the procedure is a fair one. Designing such a procedure could be left to an appropriately informed, public, democratically selected group. This is pretty much where I land in this debate.

Unfortunately, the argument does not end here (as Kamm, 1989:216–17 notes). Some philosophers (Scanlon, 1982) argue that a different standard should be used for selecting fair procedures. Scanlon argues that a procedure will count as fair when those who actually turn out to fare worst on it can have "no reasonable regrets" about the outcomes. The justification is not merely *ex ante*, from the perspective of those who share some chance of faring worst. The question then becomes whether someone who would not be chosen because another patient stands to have a better (20 year longer) outcome can have "reasonable" regrets about a procedure that selects for good outcomes. Having such regrets presumably involves rejecting the idea that the natural lottery has already exhausted the claim of equal chances. I am not sure whether reasonable regrets emerge in this case. If they do, models of justification appear to conflict.

I cannot resolve this dispute. It turns on deep theoretical disagreements about the nature of contractarian justification. The fact that these disagreements may underlie—and help explain—our uncertainty about how to resolve disputes about the acceptability of selection criteria is itself interesting. In the face of such philosophical disputes, one alternative is that we should count a procedure as fair if it is free of clearly unacceptable forms of discrimination and bias and results from the careful deliberations of a public, democractically selected group or task force (cf. Brock, 1988). But such task force deliberations leave us with the very dispute about fairness we have been discussing. We do not leave democratic, public choices immune to further testing by moral arguments.

The implications of the genome project for the distribution of scarce resources, such as organs, thus depends on how we resolve a standing dispute about patient selection criteria. Despite the fact that most people seem to favor giving weight to "best outcomes," at least to ensure a threshold of adequate outcome is reached, a fact reflected in our point systems for patient selection, the underlying moral issue remains controversial.

Are Health Risks Individual
Assets or Collective Burdens?

Suppose that one outcome of the genome project is the development of various screening tests that allow us to predict who is at higher risk for a variety of medical conditions. These tests could be used to improve what I shall refer to as standard underwriting practices (Daniels, 1990b, 1995): denying coverage, or offering more expensive and substandard coverage, to those who have a disease or are at higher risk of contracting it in the future, as determined by various medical examinations, tests, records, or other "predictors" of risk. Is there a sound moral justification for these practices?

The best strategy for insurers would be to develop a knock-down argument showing that we are morally required to use standard underwriting practices. Such an argument would seize the high moral ground and not simply rest on an appeal to their economic interest. Seeking such an argument, some insurers argue that it is actuarially unfair, and therefore morally unfair, to those at low medical risk when insurers do not exclude those at high risk from insurance pools. Thus the hybrid term, "actuarial fairness," widely used in the literature, expresses the moral judgment that fair underwriting practices must reflect the division of people according to the actuarially accurate determination of their risks. I shall refer to this as the Argument from Actuarial Fairness.

Let us begin by thinking solely about the risk-management aspect of medical insurance, ignoring for the moment any special moral importance we may attribute to assuring access to health care services. From this perspective, health insurance is only a way for rational economic agents to manage their risks of serious losses under conditions of uncertainty. Prudent people buy insurance because they prefer to face modest losses (premiums) on a regular basis rather than face catastrophic losses at unpredictable times. The absence of information about when losses will occur gives people an interest in pooling risks. When all parties symmetrically lack information, prudent consumers of insurance will have a common interest in sharing their risks.

The situation changes when we acquire information that allows us to disaggregate the risk and sort people into stratified risk pools. For example, suppose we can differentiate risks by using information about the construction, age, density and location of houses, as well as information about available firefighting facilities and relevant fire safety codes. Or suppose we can differentiate risks through information about individual medical histories, genetic disposition to disease or genetic disorders (Antonarkakis, 1989), or lifestyle choices. Then, those purchasing insurance will come to see themselves as having distinct rather than common interests. Those at lower risk will prefer to pool their risks only with others at comparably low risk, since that will lower the cost of buying security. They may not want to subsidize security for those at higher risk. At the same time, those at high risk will seek the bargain in security offered by insurance that pools high and low risk individuals (this is called adverse selection).

Insurers must respond to these consumer preferences. They must protect themselves against adverse selection, excluding those at higher risk; then they can aggressively market insurance to those at lower risk who seek security at a lower price. The behavior of insurers thus responds to competitive forces in a particular marketing context, one that assumes health insurance has the primary function of giving individuals the opportunity to manage risks prudently (Hammond and Shapiro, 1986). This assumption, as we shall see, is far from morally neutral. Changing the rules governing insurance marketing, by making insurance compulsory, for example, or by requiring that all insurance be community rated, would not eliminate the profit from insurance. But justifying those changes requires a different assumption about the function of insurance, e.g., that insurance is necessary to guarantee people adequate access to medical care.

The concept of actuarial fairness could be assigned a purely descriptive as opposed to normative content in the kind of "risk management" insurance market we have just been considering. Saying that a premium is "actuarially fair" would mean only that it reflects the actuarial risks the purchaser faces, i.e., that it is actuarially accurate. The appeal to actuarial fairness that we find in the insurance literature goes beyond this purely descriptive content, however, and carries the implication that actuarially accurate underwriting practices are also morally fair or just ones. Thus insurers defend standard underwriting practices by claiming that "Insurance is founded on the principle that policyholders with the same expected risk of loss should be treated equally. . . . The primary goal of underwriting is the accurate prediction of future mortality and morbidity costs. An insurance company has the *responsibility* to treat all its policyholders *fairly* by establishing premiums at a level consistent with the risk represented by each individual policyholder" (Clifford and Iuculano, 1987:1807–809, emphasis added). Specifically, it will be unfair to those at low risk if they are made to pay the higher premiums necessary to cover the costs of those at high risk. The remark about the "responsibility" of insurers suggests that it is an obligation to refuse to underwrite those at high risk.

The Argument from Actuarial Fairness confuses actuarial fairness with moral fairness or just distribution. These are different notions: actuarial fairness is neither a necessary nor a sufficient condition for moral fairness or justice in an insurance scheme, especially in a health insurance scheme. To forge the link this argument does between fairness and actuarial fairness presupposes that individuals are entitled to benefit from any of their individual differences, especially their different risks for disease and disability. This presupposition is not only highly controversial, it is false.

To get from the merely descriptive notion of actuarial fairness, which has no justificatory force, to the moral claim about fairness found in the insurer's argument, we need to add some moral assumptions. Specifically, we have to add the strong assumption that individuals should be free to pursue the economic advantage that derives from any of their individual traits, including their proneness to disease and disability. The strong assumption might be used in an argument that echoes some recent work on distributive justice: (1) Individual differences—any individual differences—constitute some of an individual's personal assets; (2) People should be free to, indeed, are entitled to, gain advantages from any of their personal assets; (3) Social arrangements will be just only if they respect such liberties and entitlements; (4) Specifically, individuals are entitled to have markets, including medical insurance markets, structured in such a way that they can pursue the advantages that can derive from their personal assets.

This skeletal argument can be elaborated, and the strong assumption it contains be defended (or attacked), in quite different ways within different theories of justice. For example, Nozick's libertarianism begins with certain assumptions about property rights and the degree to which certain liberties, such as the liberty to exchange one's marketable abilitites or traits for personal advantage, must be respected even in the face of what many take to be overriding social goals (Nozick, 1974). Consequently, actuarially unfair schemes confiscate property without consent. Other political philosophers claim that just arrangements are the result of a bargain made by rational people who want to divide the benefits of mutual cooperation (Gauthier, 1986). On this view, bargainers who have initial advantages in assets would only accept social arrangments that retain their relative advantages. As a result, bargainers might argue that just arrangements would preserve the advantages of those at low risk of disease through insurance markets that use standard underwriting practices.

An important objection to both libertarian and bargaining approaches is that the significant inequalities such theories justify can be traced back to initial inequalities for which there is little moral justification. To avoid this problem, Rawls imagines a "hypothetical contract" made by "free" and "equal" moral agents who are kept from knowing anything about their individual traits; they must select principles of justice that would work to everyone's advantage, including those who are worst off. Just which individual differences should be allowed to yield individual advantage thus becomes a matter for deliberation within the theory of justice, not a starting point for it (Rawls, 1971). We now need an argument why this model for selecting principles is fair to all people and why we should count its outcome as justified, since we can no longer claim they are justified by appealing to the interests of actual property holders or bargainers (Rawls, 1980, 1989).

The debate about the relevance of individual differences to the just distributions of social goods thus touches on deep issues about equality that lie at the heart of the conflict between alternative approaches to constructing and justifying theories of justice. Showing that the strong assumption about individual differences is deeply controversial at the level of the theory of justice is obviously not a refutation of the Argument from Actuarial Fairness. Still, we now have good reason not to accept the assumption without a convincing argument.

As it stands, the strong assumption is much too strong. Some individual differences are ones we clearly think should not be allowed to yield advantage or disadvantage. In recent legislation in the United States, we have established a legal framework to reinforce these views about justice. For example, we believe that race or sex should not become a basis for advantage or disadvantage in the distribution of rights, liberties, opportunities, or economic gain, even though these traits carry with them market advantage and disadvantage. Thus we reject, in its most general form, the view that all individual differences can be a moral basis for advantage or disadvantage.

Though we agree that race and sex are clearly unacceptable bases for advantage, we have less agreement about how to treat some other individual differences. We allow talents and skills, for example, to play a role in the generation of inequalities, and yet we tax those with the most highly rewarded talents and skills in ways that help those who lack them, at least to some extent (though not to the extent that the worst off are made as well off as possible, as Rawls would have it). How much inequality we allow is controversial in practice, just as it is in theory. Some people, like Nozick, think that individuals are entitled to derive whatever advantages the market allows from their talents and skills, and they view income redistribution as an unjustifiable tax on talents and skills. Others, like Rawls, argue that talents and skills, such as intelligence or manual dexterity, are the results of a "natural lottery," and that it is a matter of luck, not desert, who enjoys the family and social structures that encourage traits of character, such as diligence, necessary to refine one's basic talents. On this view, redistributive schemes are a morally obligatory form of social insurance that protects us against turning out to be among those who are worst off with regard to marketable talents and skills.

Even among those philosophers who want to treat talents and skills as individual assets, only the strictest libertarians treat health status differences merely as "unfortunate" variations and believe that there is no social obligation to correct for the relative advantages and disadvantages caused by disease or disability (Engelhardt, 1986). The design of health care systems throughout most of the world rests on a rejection of the view that individuals should have the opportunity to gain economic advantage from differences in their health risks. Despite variations in how these societies distribute the premium and tax burdens of financing universal health care insurance, our mixed system is nearly unique in allowing the degree of risks to play such a role. Moreover, surveys show that most Americans would prefer a universal system that abolished that practice. Far from being a self-evident or intuitively obvious moral principle, the strong assumption is widely rejected, both in theory and practice.

Two further points about the practice of insurers and society strengthen the claim that we do not in fact treat actuarial fairness as a basic principle of distributive justice. If insurers thought it were such a basic principle, we might expect that they would try to develop and use all possible information about variations in risk among insurees. But insurers use information about risks only when it is in *their economic interest* to do so. In effect, the principle actually underlying their practice is that we are entitled to benefit from our differences only if the market makes it profitable for insurers to provide such benefits.

This market-based entitlement can be construed as a principle of fairness only if we think the market is a fair procedure for drawing the distinctions we want to make. But, and this is the second point, we do not trust the market to draw the distinctions we think it is fair to make in this regard. We *override* appeals to actuarial fairness for many reasons in both medical and nonmedical insurance contexts. For example, we condemned "redlining" in the late 1970's as an unacceptable underwriting practice, though no one questioned its utility as a (rough) predictor of risks of loss. Similarly, unisex rating is a rejection of an actuarially fair and efficient method of underwriting and pricing groups at differential risk, but we here override standard underwriting practices because we give more importance to a principle of distributive justice assuring equal treatment of groups that are the traditional targets of discrimination. Similarly, some states have established insurance pools that guarantee no one is deemed uninsurable because of prior medical condition or high-risk classification. Where such pools are funded by insurance premiums paid by low risk individuals, we simply have an enforced subsidy from those at low risk to those at high risk, overriding concerns about actuarial fairness. Our practice—including our acceptance of Medicare and Medicaid, non-risk-rated public insurance schemes—shows that we do not believe that actuarial fairness is a basic requirement of justice.

I turn now to my main argument for rejecting the view that health insurance must be structured so that individuals can derive benefits from their differences in medical risks. Health care does many things for people: it extends life, reduces suffering, provides information and assurance, and in other ways improves quality of life. Nevertheless, it has one general function of overriding importance for purposes of justice: it maintains, restores, or compensates for the loss of—in short protects—functioning that is normal for a member of our species. Normal functioning is a crucial determinant of the opportunities open to an individual, since disease or disability shrink the range of opportunities that would otherwise have been available to someone with particular talents and skills in a given society. Since justice requires that we protect *fair equality of opportunity* for individuals in a society, it requires that we design health care institutions, including their method of reimbursement, so that they protect opportunity as well as possible within reasonable limits on resources (Daniels, 1985). Specifically, justice requires that there be no financial barriers to access to care and that the system allocate its limited resources so that they work effectively to protect normal functioning and thus fair equality of opportunity. In fact, we have a rough way to assess the importance of particular health care services, namely, by their effect on the normal opportunity range. Any general theory of justice that includes a strong principle protecting fair equality of opportunity will be able to incorporate my account of justice and health care.

The view I have been sketching involves rejecting the Argument from Actuarial Fairness. A health care system is just, provided that it protects fair equality of opportunity. Our system uses standard underwriting practices, but it fails to protect equal opportunity, since access to care depends on ability to pay. Therefore, these underwriting practices are not a sufficient condition for assuring the system is just. It will be clear from what follows that these practices are not a necessary condition either.

The most common way to try to meet social obligations regarding access to health care is to institute a universal, compulsory national health insurance scheme. Under social insurance schemes, prior medical conditions and risk classification can not serve as the basis for underwriting or pricing insurance coverage. Rather, because society acts on its obligation to meet all reasonable health care needs, within limits on resources, there will be subsidies from the well to the ill and from low risk to high risk individuals, as well as from the rich to the poor. The social insurance scheme thus requires what a private market for health insurance would condemn as actuarially unfair. This point is independent of whether the national health insurance scheme includes a sector with private insurance: The German and Dutch systems, for example, have many private insurers, but they are prohibited from using our standard underwriting practices.

From the perspective of a private insurer in our mixed system, denying coverage to those at high risk seems completely unproblematic ("You can't buy fire insurance once the engines are on the way"). But this perspective is persuasive only if the central function of health insurance is risk management. Since health insurance has a different social function, protecting equality of opportunity by guaranteeing access to an appropriate array of medical services, then there is a clear mismatch between standard underwriting practices and the social function of health insurance. A just, purely public health insurance system thus leaves no room for the notion of actuarial fairness.

Ironically, a just, but mixed public and private health insurance system makes actuarial fairness a largely illusory, perhaps even deceptive, notion. Suppose that high-risk individuals are excluded from private insurance schemes in a mixed insurance system, for the kinds of reasons we have noted earlier. Since the system is just, however, these people will not be left uninsured, as many are in the United States today. They will be covered by public insurance or by legally mandated high-risk insurance pools subsidized by premiums from private insurance. Those lower-risk individuals left in the private insurance schemes might think that actuarial fairness has protected them from higher premiums. But here is where their savings are largely illusory. The premiums of those in the private insurance schemes will either cross-subsidize the high-risk individuals who are insured in the special high-risk pools, or their taxes will cover the costs of insuring high-risk individuals through public schemes. Their actual insurance premiums are thus their private ones plus the share of their taxes that goes to public insurance.

The main point of principle in a just, mixed system is this: Low-risk individuals still share the burden of financing the health risks of high-risk individuals. Fairness requires that these risks be shared, not, as the Argument from Actuarial Fairness would have it, that they not be. In effect, health risks are not treated as economic assets and liabilities for the individual.

The genome project will generate information that insurers in our system will want to use in standard underwriting practices, not because they are greedy but because they respond to the incentives we have built into the design of our system. The argument I have offered says that such uses will make our system less fair, more unjust. But the problem is not that new information emerges from the genome project. In a national health insurance scheme that prohibited our morally unacceptable underwriting practices, information about risks would not be used to exclude people from treatment but to improve counseling, education, prevention, and treatment. It is not the availability of the information that is bad, but how our system forces us to use it. If we fail to correct the more basic injustice in the health care system, then singling out information from the genome project for special treatment would itself seem arbitrary. The problem must be corrected at its source—the design of our health care system—not simply where a new symptom of the injustice arises.

Can We Retain the Treatment/ Enhancement Distinction?

We have social obligations to treat disease and disability because of their impact on opportunity, and so we should not accept the barriers to access that follow from standard underwriting practices. Are these obligations limited to treating disease and disability? Or does any condition that creates an inequality in opportunity for welfare or advantage between individuals give rise to claims on others? In rejecting the argument from actuarial fairness, we countered an attack from the right on our social obligations to treat disease and disability. I want to consider now an attack from the left on the way I have formulated these obligations. The attack rests on the view that our egalitarian concerns require us to eliminate inequalities between persons that arise from many conditions other than disease and disability. In effect, it is a demand for a more radical version of equality of opportunity. In the context of health care, the attack takes the form of a challenge to the distinction between treatment and enhancement. If the attack is successful it has major implications for the distribution of resources, undercutting our standard way of limiting our obligations to meet individual demands for services.

I suggested earlier that the genome project may provide us with information that will erode the distinction we often draw between uses of medical technology for treatment of disease and disability and uses that enhance human appearance or performance. This distinction is closely connected to the frequently used, but poorly understood concept of "medical necessity." Many public and private insurance schemes in the United States (and Canada) claim to provide only medically necessary services: many services that involve only enhancement (e.g., cosmetic surgery) are thus excluded from coverage on these grounds. I shall suggest in what follows that the treatment/enhancement distinction does have a moral justification, at least relative to a *standard* way of thinking about equality of opportunity. The genetic information about human variation provided by the genome project may make that distinction seem more arbitrary, and to the extent that it does, it poses a challenge to the standard model and the use to which I have put it in thinking about justice and health care. Of course, this is not a conceptually novel threat: viewed from the perspective of the attack from the left, the distinction and the standard model it depends on already seem arbitrary. But the new information may heighten that appearance, and that is the reason for discussing the issue here.

Medical Need and the Scope of Obligations to Treat

Many medical technologies, new and old, can alter people in ways they desire to be changed. When do we have a social obligation to assure that such preferences are met? Do rights to health care include entitlements to have those preferences met, resources permitting? What should insurance cover?

The most inclusive answer to these questions is that we have such obligations whenever someone desires to eliminate an unwanted physical or mental condition. This would allow subjective preferences to place enormous demands on resources, holding us hostage to the extravagant tastes of others (Rawls, 1980; Dworkin, 1982). Since we do not believe it is medicine's task to make everyone equally happy, we reject this view and its implication that we should have to pay for liposuction or face lifts. Instead we think obligations arise only when medical treatments address more important problems. The stance we take about medicine is compatible with rejecting, as Rawls and Dworkin do, a broad form of egalitarianism that would require us to ensure the equal welfare or happiness of all individuals.

A less inclusive answer is that we have obligations to provide medical care whenever people desire to eliminate conditions that put them at some disadvantage. The notion of disadvantage is meant to be objective, including some forms of suffering as well as the competitive disadvantages that result from the lack of capabilities, such as marketable talents or skills. This view has some initial grip on us when disadvantages are not our fault or the result of our prior choices. Our egalitarian inclinations may incline us to think we owe something toward eliminating them (Cohen, 1989; Arneson, 1988; Sen, 1990). If we adopt such a radical view—the left position I referred to earlier—we may have to assign medicine a much greater role as a social equalizer than we now assign it. At least currently, it is not medicine's task to make everyone an equal competitor, wherever possible eliminating all inequalities in the distribution of talents and skills or other capabilities (Daniels, 1990).

A more modest answer that tends to match a wide range of our practices, including our insurance practices, is that we have obligations to provide services whenever someone desires that a medical need be met. Generally, this is taken to mean that the service involves *treatment of a disease or disability*, where disease and disability are seen as departures from species-typical normal organization or functioning (Boorse, 1977, 1975). Characterizing medical need in this way implies a contrast between uses of medical services that treat disease (or disability) conditions and uses that merely enhance human performance or appearance. Enhancement does not meet a medical need even where the service may correct for a competitive disadvantage that does not result from prior choices. Accordingly, medicine has the role of making people *normal* competitors, not *equal* competitors; this role fits, I shall claim, with the standard model for thinking about equality of opportunity.

Challenges to the Distinction

Despite its wide appeal, the distinction between treatment and enhancement seems arbitrary in light of hard cases like these:

> Johnny is a short 11-year-old boy with documented growth hormone deficiency resulting from a brain tumor. His parents are of average height. His predicted adult height without GH treatment is approximately 160 cm (5 feet 3 inches).
> Billy is a short 11-year-old boy with normal GH secretion according to current testing methods. However, his parents are extremely short, and he has a predicted adult height of 160 cm (5 feet 3 inches). (Allen and Fost, 1990)

These cases make the distinction seem arbitrary for several reasons. First, Johnny and Billy will suffer disadvantage equally if they are not treated. There is no reason to think the difference in the underlying causes of their shortness will lead people to treat them in ways that make one happier or more advantaged than the other. Second, although Johnny is short because of dysfunction whereas Billy is short because of his (normal) genotype, both are short through no choice or fault of their own. The shortness is in both cases the result of a biological, "natural lottery." Both thus seem to suffer undeserved disadvantages. Third, Billy's preference for greater height, just like Johnny's, is a preference that most people hold; it is not peculiar, idiosyncratic, or extravagant. Indeed, it is a response to a social prejudice. The prejudice is what we should condemn, not the fact that they both form an "expensive taste" in reaction to it.

Cases like these raise the following question: Does the concept of disease underlying the treatment/enhancement distinction force us to treat relevantly similar cases in dissimilar ways? Are we violating the old Aristotelian requirement that justice requires treating like cases similarly? Is dissimilar treatment unfair or unjust?

190

The Treatment/Enhancement Distinction and Equality of Opportunity

Despite the challenge of hard cases, the treatment/enhancement distinction should play a role in deciding what obligations we have to provide medical services. To show that this distinction is not arbitrary from the point of view of justice, despite the hard cases, I shall argue that it fits better with what I shall call the standard model for thinking about equality of opportunity than alternatives (Sabin and Daniels 1994). Of course, the standard model may itself be indefensible, a point I return to shortly. First I want to show that the standard model helps specify a reasonable limit on the central task of health care.

Earlier I noted that disease and disability restrict the range of opportunities open to an individual. Health care services maintain, restore, and compensate for losses of function that result from disease and disability. They thus restore people to the range of capabilities they would have had without disease or disability, given their allotment of talents and skills. Our standard model for thinking about equality of opportunity thus depends on *taking as a given the fact that talents and skills and other capabilities are not distributed equally* among people. Some people are better at some things than others. Accordingly, we assure people fair equality of opportunity if we judge them by their capabilities while ignoring "morally irrelevant" traits such as sex or race when we place people in schools, jobs, and offices. Often, however, we must correct for cases in which capabilities have been misdeveloped through racist, sexist, or other discriminatory practices. Similarly, by preventing or treating disease and disability, we can correct for impairment of the capabilities people would otherwise have. The standard model does not call for eliminating differences in normal capabilities in general, let alone through medical enhancement.

This limitation of the standard model can appear arbitrary. As I noted earlier, our capabilities are themselves the result of a natural and social lottery, and we do not "deserve" them. We just are fortunate or unfortunate in having them. We can mitigate this underlying arbitrariness somewhat as follows. Those who are better endowed with marketable capabilities are likely to enjoy more goods such as income, wealth, and power. If we constrain inequalities in these goods so that those who are worst off do as well as possible, considering all alternatives, then social cooperation will work to the benefit of all (Rawls, 1971; J. Cohen, 1988). Still, this constraint does not eliminate all inequalities in the individual capabilities or in the resulting opportunities individuals enjoy, especially since we are enjoined to judge people by their capabilities, not their "morally irrelevant" traits such as sex or race. If our egalitarian concerns require that we strive to give people equal capabilities, wherever technologically feasible, then we should not settle for mitigating the effects of the normal distribution of capabilities, as proponents of the standard model of equality of opportunity would have it (Sen, 1990). Rejecting the standard model pushes us toward equalizing all differences in capabilities; from that perspective, the distinction between treatment and enhancement has no point, at least where enhancement is aimed at equalizing capabilities.

Information from the genome project might make the distinction between disease (including genetic disease) and the normal distribution of capabilities seem more arbitrary. Suppose we learn that some particular pattern of genes explains the extreme shortness of Johnny, the child who did not seem to be growth hormone deficient. We learn, that is, just which "losing numbers" in the natural lottery placed Johnny in the bottom 1% of the normal distribution for height. Identifying these genes may then tempt us to think of them as "bad" ones: they lead to Johnny's unhappiness or disadvantage in a "heightist" world. We will then be sorely tempted to think of them very much on the model of genetic defects or diseases, especially if they work through mechanisms that have some analogy to pathological defects. We will be tempted, that is, to medicalize what we have hitherto considered normal. What, after all, allows us to treat the "bad genes" differently from genes that lead to growth hormone deficiency or to receptor insensitivity to growth hormone? If we can remedy the effects of these genes with growth hormone treatment or other treatments, including genetic tampering, we might think it quite arbitrary to maintain the treatment/enhancement distinction.

I want to offer several points as a limited defense of the standard model and the treatment/enhancement distinction (see also Sabin and Daniels, 1994, Daniels 1996). Both versions of equality of opportunity, the standard model and the more radical one that requires equalizing capabilities, seem to appeal to the same underlying intuition, that advantages and disadvantages resulting from the natural lottery are not themselves deserved. But they use the intuition differently. The standard model suggests we mitigate the effects of normally distributed capabilities through restrictions on other inequalities we allow. Since some inequality in capabilities is a fact of life, the task is to mitigate their effects while adopting principles that let everyone benefit from social cooperation. The criticism from the left rests far more weight on the underlying intuition: it says that wherever possible we must actually try to reduce variance in the distribution of capabilities, equalizing them wherever possible. I believe that the standard model better captures our actual concerns about equality than the more radical version. (Of course, our actual concerns may be too limited, so this is not a conclusive argument.)

Some supporting evidence for this point derives from our moral beliefs and practices concerning health care. We regard medical services as meeting urgent needs when they are aimed at restoring or maintaining "normal functioning." Our consensus about where to draw the line focuses on eliminating disease and disability. We already have many technologies that can enhance functioning for individuals, even giving them advantages (beauty, athletic performance) they previously did not have. But we generally resist assimilating these cases of enhancement to cases of treatment because we do not see them as meeting important needs. Although these enhancing services alter traits that may be the results of a natural lottery, they involve optimizing capabilities that are not departures from normal functional organization or functioning.

Of course, what makes the case of Billy and Johnny problematic is that they both suffer equal disadvantage as a result of the natural lottery (and social prejudice). But there is justification for adhering to a distinction that captures and sustains social agreement on important matters, even if the distinction seems arbitrary in isolated hard cases. The line between treatment and enhancement is generally uncontroversial and ascertainable through publicly accepted methods, such as those of the biomedical sciences. Being able to draw a line in this way allows us to refer in a relatively clear and objective way to the range of opportunities a person would have had in the absence of disease and disability; it facilitates public agreement. Because of these virtues, not every hard case counts as a counter-example that warrants overturning the distinction.

The "equal capabilities" approach, bolstered by new information from the genome project, is likely to undermine agreement on the importance of meeting medical needs. According to it, we would now have many more such needs, for much of what we now take to be normal would become conditions in need of rectification. Since we are far less likely to think that it is "urgent" to correct the effects of these newly labeled "bad genes," shifting away from the standard model is likely to undermine consensus on the moral importance of health care.

Will it be possible to hold the line? Some relief may come from a more careful attempt to examine the distinction between genetic disease and normal variation. This may enable us to offer a theoretical justification, coming out of the biological sciences, for a baseline distinction. It is important to note that I am not trying to save the appeal here to a natural baseline for metaphysical reasons: there is nothing magical about a natural baseline. Nor am I violating Hume's injunction against deriving 'ought' from 'is.' Rather, the natural baseline both facilitates and reflects moral agreement about the urgency of medical care. I also believe there is moral justification for limiting in some ways the task involved in protecting equality of opportunity; otherwise it will be discredited as too demanding an ideal. If, however, no theoretical justification is forthcoming that lets us distinguish "bad (or nonoptimal) genes" from genetic disease, then we will have to give more complex justifications for drawing the line between cases where we have obligations to provide services from those in which we do not. My claim is simply that it will be harder to reach consensus on these justifications without the ability to appeal to a natural baseline, however imperfectly drawn.

I have been offering reasons not to expand our goals in protecting equality of opportunity from the more limited ones of the standard model to the more encompassing one of equalizing capabilities. Nevertheless, our obligations to provide medical services need not derive solely from the concerns about equality of opportunity I have argued are central. For example, I think we have compelling reasons for providing public funding of non-therapeutic abortions that go beyond their importance for preventive health care. Similarly, suppose an inexpensive treatment became available for improving cognitive capabilities in childhood; administering it would greatly enhance the results of education, close the gap between poor but "normal" students and others, and contribute greatly to social productivity. We might then have compelling reasons to seek enhancement in this way, even if they differ from our standard justification for the importance of health care. Of course, we already have excellent reasons for putting more resources into education, yet we do not, despite the fact that our failure to do so results in misdeveloped talents and skills along race and class lines.

It might be thought that resource implications of the threat to the treatment/enhancement distinction posed by the genome project do not depend on facts about the design of our health care system. To be sure, demand for enhancement services may arise in any system, including a universal access insurance scheme that exercises strong controls over technology dissemination. But how that demand is responded to will differ depending on the nature of the system. Our system allows different insurers to adopt quite different approaches toward reimbursement for new therapies. Under some competitive pressures, it seems much more likely that some insurers in the United States would try to use coverage for enhancement therapies to achieve market advantage. The prospects are for quite unequal access to such services, followed by a general erosion of the resource constraints on enhancement technologies.

Conclusions

I have discussed three ways in which the genome project has important implications for the distribution of medical resources; two result from increased ability to predict health risks for individuals and the third results from increased ability to modify variations in human capabilities. None of these effects on resources is novel: we face all of them to some extent. Nevertheless, the genome projects makes it more urgent that we resolve the moral controversies that surround each of them. Some of the effects depend crucially on the design of our health care system, and the scope and importance of each depends on our resolving the moral disputes that underlie each of them. I have clearly raised more questions than I have answered, but seeing clearly what the questions are is a crucial first step toward answering them.

Acknowledgement: This work was in part supported by the National Endowment for the Humanities (RH20917) and the National Library of Medicine (1RO1LM05005). I have drawn on material in Daniels 1990b and Daniels 1992 in relevant sections of this paper. Publication of this paper was supported by the ELSI grant "The Genome Initiative and Access to Health Care" (1RO1HG00503-01).

References

Allen, D. B., and Fost, N. C. 1990. "Growth hormone therapy for short stature: panacea or pandora's box?" *Journal of Pediatrics*, 117:1:16–21.

Antonarkakis S. E. 1989. "Diagnosis of genetic disorders at the DNA level." *New England Journal of Medicine*, 320:153–61.

Arneson, R. J. 1988. "Equality and equal opportunity for welfare." *Philosophical Studies*, 54:79–95.

Boorse, C. 1975. "On the distinction between disease and illness." *Philosophy and Public Affairs*, 5:1:49–68.

———. 1977. "Health as a theoretical concept." *Philosophy of Science*, 44:542–73.

Brock, D. 1988. "Ethical issues in recipient selection for organ transplantation." In D. Mathieu, ed. *Organ Substitution Technology: Ethical, Legal, and Public Policy Issues*. Boulder: Westview, pp. 86–99.

Clifford, K. A., and Iuculano R. P. 1987. "Aids and insurance: The rationale for AIDS-related testing." *Harvard Law Review*, 100:1806–24.

Cohen, G. A. 1989. "On the currency of egalitarian justice." *Ethics*, 99:4:906–44.

Cohen, J. 1989. "Democratic equality." *Ethics*, 99:4:727–51.

Daniels, N. 1985. *Just Health Care*. Cambridge: Cambridge University Press.

———. 1988. "Justice and the dissemination of 'big-ticket' technologies." In D. Mathieu, ed. *Organ Substitution Technology: Ethical, Legal, and Public Policy Issues*. Boulder: Westview, pp. 211–20.

———. 1990. "Equality of what: Welfare, resources, or capabilities?" *Philosophy and Phenomenological Research*. 50 (Supplement): 273–96.

———. 1990b. "Insurability and the HIV problem: Ethical issues in underwriting." *Milbank Quarterly*, 68:4:497–526.

———. 1992. "Growth hormone therapy for short stature: Can we support the treatment/enhancement distinction?" *Growth, Genetics, and Hormones*, (Supplementary issue, in press).

———. 1995. *Seeking Fair Treatment: From the AIDS Epidemic to National Health Care Reform*. New York: Oxford University Press.

———. 1996. *Justice and Justification: Reflective Equilibrium in Theory and Practice*. New York: Cambridge University Press.

Dworkin, R. 1982. "What is equality? Part I: Equality of welfare." *Philosophy and Public Affairs*, 10:3:185–246.

Engelhardt, T. 1986. *The Foundations of Bioethics*. New York: Oxford University Press.

Gauthier, D. 1986. *Morals by Agreement*. Oxford: Oxford University Press.

Hammond, J. D., and Shapiro, A. F. 1986. "Aids and the limits of insurability." *Milbank Quarterly*, 64 (Supplement 1):143–67.

Kamm, F. M. 1987. "The choice between people: 'Common sense' morality and doctors' choices." *Bioethics*, 1:3:255–71.

———. 1989. "The report of the U.S. task force on organ transplantation: Criticisms and alternatives." *Mount Sinai Journal of Medicine*, 56:3 (May):207–20.

———. 1993. *Morality, Mortality*, vol. 1. Oxford: Oxford University Press.

Nozick, R. 1974. *Anarchy, State, and Utopia*. New York: Basic Books.

Rawls, J. 1971. *A Theory of Justice*. Cambridge: Harvard University Press.

———. 1980. "Kantian constructivism in moral theory." *Journal of Philosophy*, 77:9:515–72.

———. 1982. "Social unity and primary goods." In A. K. Sen and B. Williams, eds. *Utilitarianism and Beyond*. Cambridge: Cambridge University Press, pp. 159–86.

———. 1989. "Justice as fairness: A briefer description" (unpublished).

Sabin, James, and Norman Daniels, "Determining 'Medical Necessity' in Mental Health Practice: A Study of Clinical Reasoning and a Proposal for Insurance Policy," *Hastings Center Reports* 24:6 (November–December), 5–13.

Sen, A. K. 1990. "Justice: means versus freedoms." *Philosophy and Public Affairs*, 19:111–21.

Ten

The Human Genome Project
Its Impact on Medical Practice

Robert F. Murray, Jr.

The practice of medicine and the delivery of health care are complex, multifaceted, interdependent activities whose character and direction have been changing in recent years. The quality and quantity of the effect that the knowledge and technology of the Human Genome Project (HGP) might have on these complex activities in the next one or two decades depends on certain background information. One needs to know something about:

1. the current climate of medical practice and the way it has been changing in the U.S.;
2. the potential shape of the health care system and the ways it is likely to affect the delivery of care; and
3. the technological developments of the HGP that have the potential to influence the emphasis or direction of medical practice.

Predictions of the future shape of health care can be, at best, only a very rough guess since the number of variables that contribute to the outcome of a specific series of events usually tends to be underestimated. Furthermore, it is also next to impossible to predict what technological innovations are likely to arise during a given period that may lead to significant and unexpected developments in the diagnosis and treatment of previously incurable or unmanageable diseases.

The three points listed above serve as the nucleus around which this chapter will be presented because information bearing on them is already available. In addition, some health care providers and policy makers have considered and presented their opinions on these issues. I will also discuss some of the ethical concerns that were developed by a multidisciplinary task force on ethical issues of the Clinton White House Task Force on Health Reform in 1993. This will provide an ethical framework within which to consider the ethical acceptability of policies and actions in health care that have been influenced by the applications of technology arising from the Human Genome Project.

There are at least two other factors that might be considered in this analysis:

1. ways of communicating new information about the HGP to health care providers and policy makers; and
2. the speed with which new technologies are likely to be accepted and the degree to which they are adopted into routine medical practice.

These variables are not discussed here because there is little or no information available to estimate the influence of these determinants on the impact of the HGP in medical practice.

What is the Current Climate of Medical Practice?

One of the more dramatic changes in the way that medicine is currently being practiced and health care delivered is illustrated by the introduction and rapid increase in the number of HMOs (Health Maintenance Organizations) and PPOs (Preferred Provider Organizations) across the country.[1,2] These functional entities have been created by health care providers, often in conjunction with health insurance companies, as a means of providing more efficient and cost effective delivery and use of medical care and other health and diagnostic facilities by practitioners and patients. These means of organizing the financing and delivery of care are intended to discourage the creation of high-cost diagnostic and treatment facilities. Another major intended effect of these programs is to slow the rate of increase of the costs of health care delivery. Both of these new programs have been responsible for significant changes in the way patients get their health care and in the locus of control in the doctor-patient relationship, as well as in the options open to the patient. Some of the most important changes that have been instituted by HMOs and other managed care programs include:

1. Many, if not most, of the more recently established HMO's are profit-making entities whose major interest is in maximizing their income and minimizing their expenditures.
2. The patients choice of doctors is limited to a list of physicians who are registered with and have been found acceptable to the HMO or the PPO. This limits the freedom to choose one's physician.
3. Patient care is managed through a primary care physician, a family practitioner, pediatrician, internist or OB/GYN physician who acts as a "gate-keeper" to the services of specialists. All diagnostic tests and referrals to specialists or for emergency care must be authorized by the primary care physician. A limited number of specialists is available for diagnostic study.
4. The procedure for seeking care and treatment is carefully prescribed by the HMO/PPO. Failure to follow the procedures as prescribed may result in nonpayment by the health insurance company for services performed by the health care providers.
5. Most important, physicians are no longer the ultimate authority determining what treatment is acceptable. Administrative evaluators review the cases and determine whether diagnostic procedures and/ or therapy recommended by the physician is to be reimbursed or covered by the health insurance contract. This can include such factors as where treatment is administered, what diagnostic studies may be performed, which specialists are brought in on the case, what treatment is preferred where more than one therapy is possible, and the length of stay in hospital.

The movement toward managed care contributes to a general trend in the practice of medicine in which control of the method of delivering medical services is shifting ever more rapidly from the health care providers to those entities that provide the financing.[3] These entities—health insurance companies, for example—establish rules, restrictions, and procedures designed to take control of patient access to the system and the delivery of services within the system.

The Future of Medical Practice

The Ethics Working Group of the Clinton White House Health Care Task Force had as its major purpose to develop "Principles and Values" which were to serve as ethical underpinnings for health care reform legislation. The Working Group set forth 14 of these, from which Brock and Daniels[4,5] have highlighted the following six:

1. Universal access to equal, comprehensive benefits that meet the individual's needs over the life span;
2. A fair financing system that imposes burdens according to ability to pay and distributes burdens fairly across generations;
3. The wise allocation of resources within health care and between health care and other "goods";
4. The delivery of effective services and the avoidance of ineffective ones through the provision of high quality care;
5. A simply organized, efficiently managed system in which individual choice, personal responsibility, and professional integrity are all respected;
6. Fair procedures for making decisions and resolving disputes.

These principles can serve, at the least, as a yardstick by which to measure the extent to which any health reform proposals would attempt to create a moral and ethically ideal system of delivering health care, in the full realization that no system that might be devised could be considered perfect in all respects.

An adequately structured national health care program will provide coverage to individuals that cannot be canceled and should not be subject to restrictions or exclusions because of pre-existing "medical" conditions. In addition, cost controls would be an essential part of this system.

In the absence of certainty about the future shape of health care in the United States, the most sensible strategy is to consider what the HGP's effect might be on medical practice with respect to a range of different health care plans. At one end of that range is what some health economists would consider the optimum ethical system of health care, namely, universal coverage with a single payer system. At the other end of the range is the current system of managed care consisting of multiple, competing health insurance companies that desire to maximize their profits. They wish to be the major financiers of health care. At this writing, commercial insurance companies are aggressively promoting a variety of managed care plans. In light of that trend, this chapter will examine the possible ways that managed care, medical practice, and the HGP interact and influence one another.

Technical Innovation in Health Care through the Human Genome Project

The variety of new ways of handling DNA lend themselves to unique and more powerful ways of diagnosing genetically determined diseases.

They even make it possible to identify individuals at just about any age who are at significantly greater risk of developing a disease because they carry in their DNA a gene or genes that increase their relative susceptibility to disease significantly more than members of the general population. Since the goal of the HGP is to map the entire genome, including non-disease-related regions, when the project is complete it will be possible to diagnose *all* of the genetically determined diseases that an individual will develop before there are symptoms or signs of the condition.

If a gene has been mapped and cloned, developing a cDNA probe to specifically identify that gene makes detection of the disorder possible in humans not only from birth to death, but even after death, as well as in very early human embryos. When combined with PCR technology, this technique has been used to provide diagnoses of genetic defects at the 8 to 16 cell stage before the early human embryo has implanted in the uterine wall. This procedure raises a most ethically troublesome aspect of the application of the technology developed in the HGP since it tends to promote a "negative eugenic" solution to the control of genetically determined diseases and has the potential for undermining one of the major positive goals of medical science, namely, the treatment and/ or cure of disease. On one hand the ability to identify and eliminate embryos that will manifest genetic diseases at the pre-implantation stage means one can avoid using abortion as an option since only embryos without the offending gene would be chosen for implantation. But on the other hand, making it easier to select out these "undesirable" or "unacceptable" embryos with the potential to develop a serious genetic disease may encourage and even promote this as a way of dealing with genetic diseases, especially when no effective therapy is available. It might even have the effect of discouraging research to find effective treatments, since the elimination of mutant genes in this way reduces the "genetic load" (the number of mutant genes) in the gene pool.

This is true for diseases that may manifest themselves early in life, but is especially troublesome for conditions that are likely to be expressed under normal circumstances in middle adult life or even in old age. This raises an especially vexing ethical dilemma when one has no effective therapy to offer the patient diagnosed presymptomatically with a serious genetic disease. Based on past experience and recent surveys, there is a strong possibility that the patient will be stigmatized, so much so that it might hamper his/her employability, insurability, and even social acceptance by the other unaffected members of the community. There is also the strong possibility that patients may seek "extremes" of treatment, as already manifest in the case of the p53 gene, a cancer-associated oncogene that occurs in individuals with Li-Fraumeni Syndrome. People with the condition may also have familial occurrence of breast cancer, soft tissue sarcomas, and other tumors. Some female patients, upon finding that they have this genetic marker and a family history of breast cancer, have voluntarily subjected themselves to prophylactic bilateral mastectomy. Investigators are also searching for genes that may indicate potential susceptibility to chronic alcoholism, and other behavioral traits such as panic disorder, schizophrenia, and manic depressive psychosis. Some investigators are convinced that we will discover genetic markers indicating predisposition to and which may even be causative for homosexuality, anorexia nervosa, violence, and "criminal behavior." There is little doubt that individuals labeled as possibly predisposed to these disorders by genetic markers would suffer serious stigmatization and genetic discrimination.[6]

Medical Practice in the "Age of the Mapped Genome"

Whether health care is being delivered in the private health insurance (HMO) environment or in some one of the variations on the theme of health care reform in which health delivery companies compete for a contract to provide care in a regional or state setting, the force that provides the overall motivation in the system is an economic one. There is increasing pressure to provide those services at the lowest possible cost to the government, the employer, and the consumer. In this climate insurers ultimately are more than likely to seek out and use information that will select and eliminate or exclude purchasers of health care whose care will be most costly. Where the disorder that is driving up health care costs is a genetically determined disease, that person and his/her genetic relatives are likely either to be required to pay much higher insurance premiums or to be eliminated altogether from the pool of those who are insured. In the current health care climate evidence has been provided by Billings[7] that insurance companies are already practicing a kind of *genetic discrimination*, for example, in families where a child has cystic fibrosis. Adopting a health care reform plan similar to the one proposed by the Clinton administration[8] would avoid penalties and/or punishment for children or adults in whom genetic disease is diagnosed early in life or before symptoms appear.

The increased power of the HGP to predict illness and/or the susceptibility to illness has the strong potential to limit rather than enhance the ability of health professionals to provide care for their patients. If health reform doesn't eliminate restrictions on coverage based on the increased risk of illness and also assure universal coverage, as has been recommended by the Task Force on Genetic Information and Health Insurance in their 1993 report,[9] the number of patients with severely constrained options will substantially increase. The net effect is likely to be that patients will be denied treatment precisely for the conditions from which they are most likely to suffer. In past years physicians often got care for these patients by shifting costs of their care to other patients. Not only are third-party payers increasingly unwilling to permit cost-shifting, they want to pay less, if possible, than the actual cost of care.

A critical factor in determining whether or not equity and fairness will operate if and when there is health reform is related to the content and quality of the minimum benefits package that would make up the essential health services that would be made available to each and every citizen. This is especially important when there is concern for a patient with a chronic condition, genetic or otherwise, for which there is relatively effective management, but no effective cure. This means that the care of a person with a genetic disorder, with a potentially long life expectancy and no effective cure, would be very expensive, creating a serious economic burden on families and managed health care systems (insurance companies). The financial burden on insurers is especially heavy for relatively common disorders, e.g., cystic fibrosis in a Caucasian population.

Health Care and Medical Practice under the Current System of Managed Care

If one assumes that the map of the human genome will be developed under the current health care system there is a definite possibility, perhaps even a likelihood, that the predominant ethical effects of the HGP, at least for the short term, will be negative. This is, in part, because of the ever-increasing pressures to control the costs of delivering health care while maximizing efficiency and the profit margin. Emphasizing the cost of caring for patients whose serious genetic diseases can be predicted by using technology and information from the HGP has a major effect. It makes the patients and possibly their genetically related family members burdensome or unacceptable economic risks and probably uninsurable. On the other hand, using HGP knowledge to label patients at future risk of specific untreatable genetic diseases might promote the development of an alliance between patient and physician with the goal of protecting the patient from the social and economic harm that this information might cause.

If patients or their employers expect to be able to purchase health insurance at affordable rates they will have to find a way to keep the negative presymptomatic information that can be provided by DNA testing out of the medical records to which health insurance companies have access. This can only be done effectively with the help of their primary care physician. Under these circumstances privacy and confidentiality will become the primary value sought by the patient, since the breach of this vital protection may result in the patient's being excluded from insurance coverage and thereby relegated to a much lower quality of health care. The patient or employer might also be forced to pay exorbitantly high premiums, which often will mean that they will eventually drop their coverage. People might try to get coverage through Medicaid, but they usually will not qualify unless they are nearly economically destitute.

Jonsen suggests earlier in this volume that physicians will probably focus more intently on the patient's future, thanks to the more potent ability derived from HGP technology to identify the presence of disease-causing genes in the asymptomatic individual. However, the patient is still faced with the problem of how to deal with the need to get adequate health care without risking the loss of future financial coverage that will almost certainly be needed. If today's health care system persists, intensive efforts will have to be made to identify ethical and effective ways to protect genetic privacy and to educate health professionals so they can more effectively guard their patients' privacy. There is also the need to be able to differentiate those cases in which presymptomatic diagnosis may be beneficial from those in which it is not. The health professional, and especially the physician, will be even more strongly pressured to confront the conflict between patient confidentiality and truthtelling, especially if they are in the position of acting as an agent for the HMO or health insurance company. This is no mean challenge since, at the moment, hospital medical records are all too readily accessible to an astonishing number of people who work in hospitals.[10] With increasing amounts of diagnosis and treatment going on in ambulatory care settings, primary care physicians are increasingly likely to become the primary guardians of these vital records. Medical record information may be most successfully protected by minimizing the number of people who have access to it. Physicians may also need to change the way they respond to insurance company requests for information about applicants.

On the other hand, the greater predictive power of human genome medicine may justify the threat to privacy *if* the predictive knowledge or information is accompanied by reasonably effective ways to treat the conditions identified, or to prevent their pathological manifestations. So if, as predicted by Polvino and Anderson in their discussion of gene therapy (see chapter 3), the HGP produces technology enabling physicians to fully and permanently correct a presymptomatic genetic defect, the risk of loss of privacy and of being labeled and/or stigmatized as inferior or inadequate, for most patients, will be more than justified by the potential benefit of having the disorder corrected. This use of HGP technology is considered a cost-effective benefit of gene mapping, to be encouraged and promoted. Unfortunately, it is likely that only a minority of genetically determined conditions will lend themselves to the ready use of this technology as it is currently conceived. On the other hand, there is no assurance that successful gene therapy (where the abnormal or deficient function is normalized) will provide a permanent cure. Thus far successful gene therapy has not been permanent, even though in theory it could be.

What HGP Technology Will be Covered?

One of the biggest questions raised by the application of HGP technology in today's managed health care climate is, "What services or therapies will be covered by insurance plans?"

One area of HGP knowledge which has generated considerable controversy is the use of genetic markers that are associated with an increased risk of serious disease, especially breast or colon cancer. These markers, such as the p53 mutants, may provide the opportunity for more aggressive case finding in families in which these markers are inherited. But such markers also occur in the population at large and offer a similar opportunity in a small minority of the population to identify high-risk individuals. Will HMOs pay for screening tests for these or other markers that may identify susceptibility to alcohol or other drug abuse? Health insurance companies have been reluctant in the past to pay for screening tests unless there is a definitive therapeutic payoff.[11] It is likely that there are genetic markers that will delineate groups of patients at increased risk to develop specific behavioral disorders, e.g., manic depressive psychosis, panic disorder or schizophrenia. Still other HGP knowledge has the potential to provide useful information to patients to help them avoid or prevent treatable conditions. These tests might be inaccessible because the technology is unproven and health insurance companies (HMOs) refuse to pay because the tests haven't been shown to be cost effective and because patients can't afford to pay for the tests.

Increasingly, physicians will be placed in the more sensitive position of "double agent," in which they will have to decide whether they owe their primary allegiance to the patient, as in the past, or to the HMO which pays their fees or salary.[12] It is fast approaching the situation where health insurance of managed care groups is by far the major source of income of physicians. Physicians whose practice style is rejected by the HMO may not be able to practice. If the HMO plays the primary role in delineating the boundaries in patient care, physicians may find it easy to yield decisions about patient privacy and autonomy to the managed care administrators.

Health Reform, Ethics, and the Human Genome Project

Even if a program of health reform were to be adopted which emphasized universal coverage and included a minimum benefit package that included genetic services, e.g., newborn screening, prenatal diagnosis, and limited presymptomatic diagnosis, some of the same ethical conflicts would face the physician if a major emphasis continued to be on competitiveness and financing by multiple insurance contractors. The program would provide for payment for all patients, but there would still be pressure to reduce costs by excluding chronically ill patients, who might be relegated to special or high-risk care groups or receive less than optimum care. In this type of system the severity of the psychosocial and/or economic consequences of being identified as a presymptomatic carrier of an autosomal dominant condition would be reduced if the health care resources of the system were readily available to the patient. Even if a significant amount of psychosocial harm is negated by the available therapeutic health benefits, one cannot avoid the potential for compromising the patient's employment opportunities. Furthermore, it is possible that specially-constituted health organizations bidding for a patient services contract would be especially motivated to exclude those individuals with potential chronic, incurable conditions, in an effort to improve their efficiency and the cost effectiveness of delivering care to patients in a particular locale. Once again the tension between doctor and patient would increase, since reducing the costs of delivering services will always be a major factor when competition in the marketplace is part of the health care equation. This factor will always create an ethical dilemma for physicians when they are faced with improvements in technology that will make it possible to identify increasing numbers of individuals at risk to develop serious genetically determined diseases for which there is little or no effective treatment. This is especially true for physicians whose income depends on the financial success of the health care network.[13] They would still be in the position of having to withhold some health care information if they wanted to reduce the harm that the technological advance might cause their patient if it were reported to the HMO. Only when knowledge of specific presymptomatic genetic markers is also associated with the ability to provide:

1)   prevention of the manifestations of disease,
2)   effective treatment for the condition, or
3)   methods to correct or cure the defect through gene therapy

can one be confident that the ethical balance will clearly be on the benefits side of the risk-benefit equation and that the focus of the benefits of medical practice would be squarely on the patient.[14]

If it were possible to choose a system of medical practice and health care delivery to minimize the harm that might come of the medical application of HGP technology, one might choose a medical system like those currently in use in most other industrialized countries, namely, *universal health care insurance under a single payer–government controlled system.* This system would be designed so as to minimize patient exploitation. In this system there would not be a health care penalty for being at risk for some future chronic disease and the combined resources of the nation would be available to provide the high-technology therapy that would be available. With no penalty for reporting the patient's disease, the physician would be free from the truthtelling/withholding dilemma and the patient would not be an "insurance outcast," with the associated stigmatization. Only properly crafted and enacted legislation could protect the patient from the negative socioeconomic consequences of the genetic label indicating that he or she is at risk of or presymptomatic for genetic disease. There would be some negative consequences of adopting this health care format. Many if not most of the financial incentives that currently exist for physicians, especially those in certain subspecialties, would be lost and the highly profitable pharmaceutical industry would be constrained in its earnings. But the major *negative effect* on patients is that hard decisions would have to be made to determine who would have access to expensive procedures such as gene therapy. It would not likely be determined by the ability to pay but, perhaps, by criteria more related to age (younger patients might get preference) and severity of condition. Limitations on the ability to choose one's physician would probably not change. But such a system would be more just than one in which socioeconomic status, influence, and financial wherewithal were the primary factors determining who got care and who didn't.

No matter what system of health care is available, the medical application of HGP technology will have a significant effect on the ethical tensions and certain of the procedures followed in the practice of medicine as we know it. But what is most important will be the processes that are established to see that diagnostic techniques that derive from the HGP are not introduced until legal and ethical protections for the patient are established, along with the means by which those harms that occur can be rectified quickly and fairly. If this is done the traditional emphasis of medical practice on the welfare and well-being of the patient can be maintained and strengthened.

Summary

The manner in which health care is delivered is already having a profound effect on the practice of medicine. The major issue that confronts health care workers is what system of health care delivery we will finally have when the economic discussions and the political debates have concluded.

Ultimately, the kind of health care system we may have may range from one like the HMOs, which feature managed care and open competition, to one like other industrialized nations featuring universal access and a single payer (most probably the federal government or its representative) or some combination of these extremes. No matter which system is adopted, information provided by HGP technology will, if prematurely introduced, create serious ethical conflicts and tensions between patients, physicians, and insurance payers if managed care continues to be emphasized. If the health care system emphasizes the needs of patients, socioeconomic problems may predominate. If HGP technology and its diagnostic and predictive information is introduced into medical practice in conjunction with effective treatment, so that it emphasizes benefit to patients, it is most likely to have a positive ethical impact consistent with justice and beneficence.

Notes

1. Iglehart, J. K., "The American health care system: Introduction." New England Journal of Medicine, 326:962–67, 1992.

2. Iglehart, J. K., "The American health care system: Managed care." New England Journal of Medicine, 327:742–47, 1992.

3. Iglehart, J. K., "Physicians and the growth of managed care." New England Journal of Medicine, 331:1167–71, 1994.

4. Daniels, N., "The articulation of values and principles involved in health care reform." Journal of Medicine and Philosophy, 19:425–33, 1994.

5. Brock, D., and N. Daniels, "Ethical foundations of the Clinton administration's proposed new health care system." Journal of the American Medical Association, 271:1189–96, 1994.

6. Billings, P. R., M. A. Kohn, M. de Cuevo, J. Beckwith, J. S. Alper, M. R. Natowicz, "Discrimination as a consequence of genetic testing." American Journal of Human Genetics, 50:476–82, 1992.

7. Starr, P., "The framework of health care reform." New England Journal of Medicine, 329:1666–71, 1993.

8. Kaiser Commission on the Future of Medicaid, *Health Reform Legislation: A Comparison of Major Proposals*, Kaiser Health Reform Project. Henry J. Kaiser Family Foundation, 1994.

9. NIH-DOE Working Group on Ethical, Legal, and Social Implications of Human Genome Research, *Genetic Information and Health Insurance*, NIH, National Center for Human Genome Research, 1994.

10. Siegler, M., "Confidentiality in medicine—A decrepit concept." New England Journal of Medicine, 307:1518–21, 1982.

11. Holtzman, N., "What drives neonatal screening programs?" New England Journal of Medicine, 325:802–804, 1991.

12. Rodwin, M. A., "Conflicts in managed care." New England Journal of Medicine, 332:604–607, 1995.

13. Ibid.

14. Institute of Medicine, Division of Health Sciences Policy, Committee on Assessing Genetic Risks, "Genetic Testing and Assessment in Assessing Genetic Risks." Washington, D.C.: National Academy Press, 59–115, 1994.

Eleven

The Genome and Access to Health Care
Two Key Ethical Issues

Thomas H. Murray

I want to discuss two major categories of ethical issues relating to access to health care prompted by the Human Genome Project. The issues are not utterly novel; indeed, if they were, it is unclear how we would have any way of articulating them or of knowing how to begin to think about their ethical ramifications. But the HGP, in each case, provides some new impetus or urgency to the question.

The first category is justice. How will new genetic technologies be allocated? Will the allocation of other services, for example transplantable organs, be affected by genetics? Will genetic prediction be used more broadly to determine who has access to health insurance?

The second major category is the distinction between therapy and enhancement. Under the press of new findings about the genetic basis of human characteristics, will we be able to sustain the distinction between the use of medical technologies for therapeutic purposes and the use of the same or related technologies in order to enhance an individual's characteristics? Should we maintain that distinction?

Each of the ethical questions raised about access in the context of the Human Genome Initiative must be examined in the light of probable changes in the structure of health care in the United States, including the increasing pressures to contain costs and the movement toward managed care. The HGP itself is likely to influence that structure: it may affect the Who Provides?, the What?, and the To Whom?, as well as the At Whose Expense? Though we cannot be anywhere near certain about what precise changes will occur, we can be reasonably sure that there will be substantial changes.

The Human Genome Project itself will not be the most important source of structural change in the United States health care system. Rather, it will interact with other forces that have provided the political impetus to alter drastically the organization and financing of health care. It is important when thinking about the effects of the HGP on access to realize that the health care system into which the fruits of the HGP will go may be dramatically different in crucial respects from the system we now have. I cannot begin to pretend to understand all of the factors influencing that transformation. But in a book on the HGP and access to health care, we must remain mindful of the other important forces while we focus explicitly on the impact of the HGP itself. Albert R. Jonsen's study of the remapping of the physician-patient relationship is a good place to begin.

Remapping the Patient-Physician Relationship

Jonsen's meditation on the impact of the Human Genome Project on the relationship between physician and patient is a useful reminder that the Genome Project will yield more than new kinds of medical information and clinical tools. It may in fact alter the system into which that information and those tools will be injected. It may change patients' self-perceptions and expectations; it may alter physicians' self-conceptions and their practice, and those changes will not be limited to clinical geneticists; it may lead to genetic information and services being delivered by new professionals in new settings—especially primary care environments; and it may alter societal beliefs and moral commitments about the cause, prevention, and treatment of disease, as well as the responsibility for health and disease borne by individuals and society.

Patients' self-perceptions and expectations. For good or ill, as genetic predictors of disease become cheap, accurate, and widely available, people will increasingly come to see themselves as the person-who-is-well-at-the-moment-but-who-is-at-risk-of . . . (or alternatively, they may think of themselves as having genetic protection against one or more diseases). It also seems likely that they will regard genetic predispositions as immutable aspects of their identity. People may perceive that genetic risks in some way constitute fundamental aspects of the self, perhaps far more fundamental than such accidentals of life as one's education, residence or work.

The self has always been shaped by and imbedded in family. But now genetic disease and disease risks form powerful links of physical continuity between the self and one's ancestors and descendants. It may be reassuring to know that your cholesterol level and consequent risk of heart disease has more to do with the genes for liver metabolism that you inherited from your parents than it does with your diet or exercise patterns. Or you may experience it as a family curse. But it seems unlikely to have no effect at all on how you think about your own health, as well as your genetic connections with your family.

In addition to its impact on self perceptions and relations with one's biological family, people's expectations about their health professionals are likely to change. Jonsen argues persuasively that medicine will return, at least in significant part, to being a *scientia contemplativa* from its current role as a *scientia activa*. Physicians—or the professionals who assume some of their current duties—may function somewhat less as intervenors and more as prognosticators, advisors, and monitors. Your physician, for example, may offer predictions about your future, telling you that you carry the recently discovered colon cancer gene. That physician then may advise you as to what you can do to reduce your risks, such as modifying your diet. The physician may also become an active monitor of your health—working with you regularly to detect signs of precancerous changes in your colon, or the first, early warnings of cancer itself. None of these tasks are entirely new to the physician. The Human Genome Project, however, may tilt physicians' work in the direction of prediction and prevention. Perhaps we will go to the doctor not merely when we are sick, but in order to learn what we are likely to become sick from and what we can do to remain healthy.

Physicians' self-conceptions and practices. Jonsen argues that therapeutic activism will give way, at least in part, to interactions that resemble those that occur between genetic counselors and their clients. The interactions will center on the exchange of information rather than focusing on interventions. The sociologist Charles Bosk, in a recently published study of clinical geneticists, offers some observations that might foretell certain changes in medicine more generally. Bosk reports that physician-geneticists distinguish sharply between the services they provide—largely the provision of information—and the work of the "green coats"—their interventionist physician colleagues in, for example, the ICUs. There are clear differences in prestige and professional identity between the interventionists and the information providers. Even fur-

Thomas H. Murray

ther down the pecking order are the professionals who deal with the emotional repercussions of genetic information. The physician-geneticists prefer to leave that messy sort of work to non-MD counselors.[1] It is interesting to speculate on what will happen if and when physicians find themselves doing what their clinical genetics colleagues have typically done. Will it lead to a general diminution in prestige for physicians? Will it lead to more balanced relationships among specialists? Will it further increase the social distance between interventionist specialists and non-interventionist primary care providers? Will physicians try to off-load the information provision to non-MDs, in much the way that the geneticists in Bosk's study off-loaded the low-prestige, emotionally trying, and time-consuming work of genetic counseling?

Any genome-inspired move by physicians to emphasize their role as information providers would deepen further a struggle between the procedure-oriented, interventionist specialties and the information and conversation-intensive forms of medical practice. Physicians who cut and probe and image earn considerably more than their colleagues who listen and watch; they also command greater prestige and power. A technique for reimbursing physician services called the Resource Based Relative Value Scale, or RBRVS, could restore a measure of balance: applying the RBRVS results in lower payments to interventionists and higher payments (in theory at least) to non-interventionist physicians. With ever-increasing pressure to reduce health care costs, it will be interesting to see if in fact the income gap between interventionists and non-interventionists narrows; whether that narrowing is accompanied by a move toward more equal power and prestige; and, if such an equalization occurs, whether physicians become more willing to take on the many non-interventionist tasks the Human Genome Project is likely to create.

New professionals in new settings? The same forces that have shaped the current debate over health care reform—principally a desire to lower the cost of health care and a concomitant belief that current incentives promote an oversupply of specialty care and an undersupply of primary care—may lead to new professionals providing genetic services in new settings.

Genetic counselors emerged as a profession that filled a gap. They understood genetics much better than most primary care physicians (whose medical education until very recently paid little or no attention to clinical genetics). Genetic counselors were trained and willing to do the sometimes messy, time-consuming work of talking, listening, and helping people cope with the emotional turmoil caused by bad genetic news. Their services also cost substantially less than physicians' services.

The desire to save money, the reluctance of many physicians to give the time or endure the emotional anguish of dealing with the aftermath of bad genetic news, and the relatively small number of trained genetic counselors combine to create a need for professionals who can do the work of communicating genetic news and dealing with the responses to it. Perhaps the number of genetic counselors will increase rapidly. Perhaps primary care physicians will embrace these tasks, although this seems unlikely without a much greater rearrangement of incentives than seems politically feasible, accompanied by a dramatic change in the recruitment and training of physicians to favor humanistic rather than technical skills. Or perhaps new tasks will be given to existing groups of health professionals, for example nurse practitioners, or new specializations may be created—genetic counselors who focus on presymptomatic or predisposition testing.

The most probable scenarios take a good deal of the work of genetic information provision and counseling away from physicians and give it to other professionals. An adequate analysis of the ethical issues involved will have to be much broader than "medical" ethics narrowly construed as the ethics of patient-physician interaction. It will have to encompass a broad range of health professional–patient interactions. It may even need to abandon the presumption that the morally most important interactions are those with physicians.

Genetic disease and responsibility. At first glance, it appears that finding a genetic cause for a disease would diminish the inclination to say that persons who develop the particular disease bear responsibility for their own plight. Albert R. Jonsen's discussion of the remapping of the patient-physician relationship suggests that the Human Genome Project instead might increase perceived individual responsibility for disease. The logic is fairly straightforward. Genetic prediction is a kind of forewarning. When an event is foreseeable, we have the responsibility to do what we reasonably can to avoid bad consequences. For certain genetically predicted diseases, we may be able to monitor ourselves for early signs and take preventive measures, or by taking care, for example, in diet and exercise, we might be able to substantially reduce risks. By bringing the future into the present, and by making the possible actual, we may increase the perception that people are responsible for their own afflictions.

This would not be irrational or morally indefensible if in fact people's diligent health care and personal habits could protect them from disease. In reality, the picture is likely to be much more ambiguous, with some proven or merely suspected measures one can take to prevent a genetically predicted disease from occurring, but where disease will strike people no matter how careful they are.

One of the ironies of increased links between genes and disease is that however the question about individual behavior is settled, perceived societal responsibility could be reduced. If on the one hand, particular diseases or diseases in general come to be seen as largely genetic, those who were reluctant to take care of their fellows in need could argue that society did not cause the person's illness, bad genes did, and that therefore society had no obligation to remedy a problem it did not cause. On the other hand, the more forewarned, and the more individuals can do to prevent disease, the more society may be inclined to declare that those individuals are responsible for their own misfortune and that the community has no obligation to step in with assistance.

Society may in contrast continue to treat ill health as something to which the community should respond. But there is nothing intrinsic about genetic causality of disease that assures that society will respond compassionately. Another feature of genetic predisposition to disease, however, may help promote the move to a health system that embraces all members of the community. But that is an issue of justice.

Issues of Justice

Questions about justice related to the Human Genome Project and access to health care take three forms in the studies that comprise this volume. There is the problem of allocating genetic services; of using genetic information to determine the allocation of other health services; and the use of predictive genetic information in health insurance underwriting.

Allocating genetic services. Maxwell J. Mehlman, in his study of access to health care in the context of federal entitlement programs, paints a bleak portrait (see chapter 6). Mehlman describes strategies used in programs such as Medicaid and Medicare to delay or deny coverage for health care technologies. In practice, a very important dividing line in access to health care has been between those with private insurance and those whose access comes through federal entitlement programs. (Another important division is between those with coverage of any kind and the roughly forty million with no coverage.) Private insurance is typically much more generous than federal programs. Mehlman imagines a near future when highly effective—and very expensive—genetic technologies become available. As long as a two-tiered system of health care coverage operates, people with generous—read "private"—insurance will gain access to these technologies, while those dependent on federal entitlement programs will find access delayed or denied. Herbert Nickens reminds us that in such a tiered system, those who lose out will be disproportionately members of minority groups (chapter 4).

To the extent that this split between private and public modes of access to health care survives the current efforts at reform, and to the extent that genetic services do emerge as effective, Mehlman worries that the differences in access could lead to intense and persistent struggle. In an especially poignant phrase, he notes that abortion could "become the poor person's gene therapy." He also is concerned that the line between genetic therapy and genetic enhancement will be difficult to sustain, that the well-off will use enhancement technologies, and that a "genetic underclass"—dependent on federal entitlement programs for their health care—will emerge.

Mehlman's dystopic scenario serves as a powerful warning that problems in justice are as—perhaps more—likely to arise if the Human Genome Project is a success than if it is a failure. That, after all, makes eminent sense: there could be no sensible struggle over access to technologies that confer no benefits. Only when the technologies are instrumental to achieving desirable goals (or avoiding burdens) do genuine questions of distributive justice arise. It seems odd to say that the best reassurance one could give Mehlman is that the Human Genome Project is unlikely to create any new, desirable technologies. But such a reassurance is almost surely false. A much better form of reassurance would be radical reform of the health care system that would provide equivalent access for all. Such a reform could ameliorate or eliminate injustice in access to genetic therapies. It would respond to the grave concerns expressed by several authors in this volume. Even if we were successful in assuring a rough measure of justice in access to health care, the problem of what to do with genetic enhancement technologies would remain.

It is unlikely, and probably unwise, for any health care system to provide genetic enhancement technologies as a part of its standard benefit package. If such technologies are developed at all, they are likely to be available on a market basis to those who desire and can afford them. Designing strategies for access to such enhancement technologies— which may amount to strategies for tight control or prohibition—could emerge as an enormously difficult policy challenge. Our recent efforts at controlling an early genetic "enhancement"—human Growth Hormone for non–hGH deficient children—is neither wholly discouraging nor encouraging.

Using genetic differences to allocate other health services. Norman Daniels, in this volume, discusses whether it is permissible to use predictive genetic information when allocating health-related goods such as life-prolonging transplantable organs. He shows that the problem is separable into at least two components: first, whether using genetic differences to allocate resources such as organs is morally defensible per se, and second, what would be entailed in constructing a fair procedure for deciding whether to allow consideration of genetic differences. Neither problem, he correctly notes, has a universally acceptable solution.

Genetic differences already count for a great deal in the allocation of some organs. HLA or antigen matching is used in the UNOS point system for allocating organs, and is entirely genetically derived. Presumably, it predicts the likelihood and intensity of rejection of the foreign organ by the host's immune system. The only arguments that tend to be raised against using HLA matching question its technical validity—that is, whether a better antigen match actually attenuates rejection—not that there is anything intrinsically "unfair" about using a genetic factor in organ allocation.

HLA matching, or course, would not be a disadvantage across all potential donor organs unless there was something about this person's or this group's antigen pattern that made it less likely to match not just one organ but the available supply as a whole. In fact, something like that happens. African Americans are less likely to be donors than other Americans, and there is some evidence of population differences in HLA antigen patterns such that organs from donors of European descent are more likely to match potential recipients with similar ethnic backgrounds. The net result of this presumably morally neutral use of a genetic difference in the pursuit of efficiency is that Americans of African descent are less likely to receive a transplant.

Should the democratic task force that Daniels prefers, composed of members who do not know how they come out in the "natural lottery," be concerned to develop a procedure that is fair not merely to individuals but to populations that display genetic differences? To avoid heaping injustice upon injustice, it appears the task force would have to take such genetic differences among populations into account.

Genetics and access to health insurance. One of the principal ways in which genetic information may be used, unless public policies are devised to provide otherwise, will be for insurance underwriting. A national task force was formed by the Ethical, Legal, and Social Issues Program of the Human Genome Project to examine the issue of genetic information and insurance and to suggest policies that would promote good uses of genetic information without the negative consequences of genetic discrimination. The task force was formed in May 1991. Its membership included representatives of the insurance industry, genetic disease groups, and other experts. Insurance representatives included the Health Insurance Association of America, the American Council of Life Insurance, and the National Blue Cross Blue Shield Association. Genetic disease group representatives included persons from the Alliance of Genetic Support Groups, the Federation for Children with Special Needs, and the Tourette Syndrome Association. The group delivered its findings in May 1993.

The task force chose to concentrate on health insurance rather than life or disability income insurance for two reasons. First, the crisis in health care, with tens of millions of Americans uninsured at any time, and with some 60 million without insurance for at least part of the year, posed an urgent social problem. Second, adverse selection—in which customers who purchase insurance know more than they reveal to insurers and are more likely to file a claim—is a less acute financial problem in health care insurance than in life or disability income insurance.

The United States health insurance system is built on a kind of catch-22—the more likely you are to need care for a particular disease, the more difficult it will be to obtain coverage for that care. Genetic prediction of disease sharpens and broadens the public perception of that catch-22. It sharpens it by making it crystal clear that a genetic disease—a disease for which the person cannot be said to bear any responsibility whatsoever—can nonetheless deprive one of any opportunity to buy affordable health insurance. It broadens it because anyone can have a genetic predisposition without knowing it, yet could have that disposition revealed by the next genetic test to be developed. None of us are more than one short step away from being at risk of genetic discrimination.

The task force made two important findings that shaped its recommendations. First, after a sustained and fruitless effort to show the morally and practically relevant differences between genetic and non-genetic information in health insurance, the task force concluded that such a distinction was morally indefensible and practically unfeasible. Morally, the central point about access to health care was that health care ought to be available to those who need it. Whether the need was a product of genetics or bad luck or other factors did not distinguish the cases where people should have access from the cases where they should not.[2]

Even if one accepted the claim that people are in some substantial way responsible for their ill health, it does not follow that those at genetic risk are morally distinct. For one thing, as described above, showing that one has a genetic predisposition to a disease does not absolve one for responsibility for one's illness. Though there are and will continue to be genetic diseases we can do nothing to prevent or cure, most of the diseases for most people will be preventable to some degree. If a person is found to be at increased genetic risk for heart disease, for example, we can expect that person to be careful about diet, exercise, weight, smoking, and other behaviors and characteristics known to affect the risk of heart disease. On the other side, there are many illnesses and accidents for which people have as little responsibility as inheriting a gene for Huntington's. Personal responsibility, per se, does not distinguish genetic from non-genetic diseases.

Suppose that we accepted a part of the claim: that people who bring on their own ill health should expect to bear some burden for it. It does not follow that diminishing their access to health care is a reasonable response. First, more often than not, it is hard to tell whether or to what extent a particular individual is responsible for his or her plight. Being 20 percent over your ideal weight may increase your risk of heart disease, but I cannot say to any particular individual that *your* heart attack is *your own* fault. It might just as well be true that this individual would have had a heart attack at the identical age if she or he had maintained the prescribed weight. Most of the risks likely to be identified by genetic testing, certainly the risks for common diseases, will be probabilistic, not deterministic.

Second, there is a very poor correlation between the offense and the "punishment"—that is, between less than perfect health habits and illness. Some people who do everything wrong health-wise nonetheless enjoy long life and good health, while others who scrupulously adhere to healthy habits are afflicted with disease. Third, most analyses of justice in health care presume that need for care is the crucial morally relevant factor, not desert. Fourth, as a matter of policy, it makes much more sense to impose taxes or other burdens on the unhealthy behavior than it does to deny health care to those who became ill in part, perhaps, by their own hand. Rather than requiring that fault be assigned, as in a civil damage suit, it would be far simpler—and more humane—to tax cigarettes, for example, than to deny palliative care to someone dying of lung cancer. Personal responsibility for illness is a poor basis on which to allocate health care; in any event, it does not mark off genetic from non-genetic diseases.

The second important finding made by the task force was that genetic tests are only a part, at this time a small part, of available genetic information. The health history, which reveals details of family member's illnesses, is a rich source of genetic information which could be used to deny insurance coverage. An exclusive focus on genetic tests would miss most of the opportunities for genetic discrimination.

Insurers argued, correctly, that there was little or no use of genetic tests at this time, and that they did not expect to see widespread use of such tests in the immediate future. But it is important to see what these claims do *not* mean. They do not mean that there is no genetic discrimination. To the contrary, insurers admit and defend their use of genetic information (from health records or health histories or the like) that has actuarial validity. They describe such use of genetic information as "fair" discrimination, in keeping with the principles of insurance underwriting as analyzed in this volume by Deborah Stone (chapter 7). They also do not mean that they will never seek to use genetic tests in underwriting. The principle reason genetic tests are not used today is that they are not believed to be cost-effective. Once the price of tests drops, as seems certain, and the actuarial data on the tests' predictive abilities accumulates, the tests will become cost-effective and therefore attractive to insurers.

The task force concluded that the only feasible and defensible way to assure that widespread genetic discrimination in health care coverage did not emerge was to reform radically the United States health care system. The task force's conclusions were as follows:

> In anticipation of fundamental reform in the financing and delivery of health care in the U.S., the Task Force on Genetic Information and Insurance offers the following recommendations. The recommendations concern health care coverage and should not be applied uncritically to other forms of insurance, such as life or disability income insurance.

> 1. Information about past, present or future health status, including genetic information, should not be used to deny health care coverage or services to anyone.

> 2. The US health care system should ensure universal access to and participation by all in a program of basic health services* that encompasses a continuum of services appropriate for the healthy to the seriously ill.

> 3. The program of basic health services should treat genetic services comparably to non-genetic services, and should encompass appropriate genetic counseling, testing and treatment within a program of primary, preventive and specialty health care services for individuals and families with genetic disorders and those at risk of genetic disease.

4. The cost of health care coverage borne by individuals and families for the program of basic health services should not be affected by information, including genetic information, about an individual's past, present or future health status.

5. Participation in and access to the program of basic health services should not depend on employment.

6. Participation in and access to the program of basic health services should not be conditioned on disclosure by individuals and families of information, including genetic information, about past, present or future health status.

7. Until participation in a program of basic health services is universal, alternative means of reducing the risk of genetic discrimination should be developed. As one step, health insurers should consider a moratorium on the use of genetic tests in underwriting. In addition, insurers could undertake vigorous educational efforts within the industry to improve the understanding of genetic information.

[*We use the phrase "program of basic health services" to describe the array of services that would be available to all after implementation of major health policy reforms, such as those being considered by the President's Health Policy Task Force. We explicitly reject all connotations of "basic" as minimal, stingy, or limited to such services as immunization and well child care. A program of "basic" health services could encompass a broad range of care for those most in need.]

Can We Sustain the Distinction between Therapy and Enhancement? Should We?

For Maxwell J. Mehlman, the prospect of genetic enhancements poses a profound threat to justice and peace. It is worth recalling his words in some detail:

Genetically enhanced individuals will gain overwhelming advantages over the non-enhanced. Equal opportunity will disappear . . . upward mobility for those without access to enhancement services will become a thing of the past. The result will be . . . a society divided between those with access to the genome and a genetic underclass . . . permanently enslaved to their genetic endowments. . . . Eventually, the degree of disparity will dwarf the social distinctions that characterized feudalism, the caste system in India, and even human slavery.[3]

Mehlman's dystopic vision is terrifying to be sure. It is also not entirely unrealistic. But it is premised on a set of empirical predictions—scientific and political—some of which are plausible and some, fortunately, less so.

Mehlman is on very solid ground when he predicts that genetic enhancements are unlikely to be included under any federal entitlement program. They are also unlikely to be paid for by private insurers, both because they are likely to be expensive and because insurers fear what is called, aptly in this instance, moral hazard—roughly the capacity of the insured to generate claims at will by, for example, burning down one's business—or embarking on a course of genetic enhancement. Genetic enhancements, should they become available, are most likely to be distributed by the market, openly or otherwise. The concerns Mehlman expresses are as relevant to a market for enhancement technologies as they would be if distributed within a multi-tiered health system.

A second prediction is that genetics will in fact become capable of offering enhancements that are socially advantageous and for which the risks are low enough that a prudent person would be willing to accept them in order the gain the potential benefit. This is certainly a possibility—the world's literature after all is littered with informed, learned commentary proving that something we now take for granted could never be done. But in fact the enhancement technologies now available are meager, with human Growth Hormone (hGH) the best known one. Nonetheless, the experience with hGH should give us pause as there is considerable anecdotal evidence that parents do seek the advantages increased height can bring for their non-hGH-deficient children.

What may save us at least in the short run is the likelihood that the complex traits that are most valued in human beings—intelligence, creativity, sociability, leadership, and the like—have the most tenuous relationship to genetics. To the extent that these humanly valued traits are genetic at all, the genetic links are complex, buried many layers beneath the environmental and developmental forces that shape them. Efforts to enhance such traits genetically will probably turn out to be fruitless, at least for the foreseeable future.

A third presumption underlying Mehlman's dystopia is that society will become increasingly unable to distinguish between what is genetic therapy and what is genetic enhancement, so that we will eventually abandon the effort to draw any line between the two. What matters most here are the public policy implications: if we cannot sustain the distinction, we cannot maintain a public policy that discourages potentially divisive and destructive markets for enhancement.

No one can say for certain whether that distinction can be held secure against challenges. Norman Daniels offers some hope that it can be and some reason that it should. Daniels begins by pointing out that a reasonably drawn distinction between therapy and enhancement does a reasonable job of capturing our moral intuitions about the limits of our obligations to provide for the needs of others. On this understanding, a therapy is a response to a genuine need, while an enhancement may be a thing people desire greatly but do not actually need. Daniels ties this observation into his theory that views health care as a means by which people's diseases and disabilities are responded to by society so that the individuals may be brought into the range of normal functioning. Once within this normal range of functioning, each person has fair equality of opportunity which, in Daniels's theory and in common sense morality, is just.

Daniels also notes the virtues of being able to draw a line, such as the one between therapy and enhancement. Such a line "allows us to refer in a relatively clear and objective way to the range of opportunities a person *would have had* in the absence of disease and disability; it facilitates public agreement" (this volume, chap. 9). He argues that the notion of a baseline of health below which is the realm of therapy and above which is the kingdom of enhancement "facilitates and reflects moral agreement about the urgency of medical care." Finally, he asserts the need to limit the scope of our obligations to protect equality of opportunity, lest it "be discredited as too demanding an ideal" (ibid.).

Defenders of a complex, morally weighty, and practically relevant distinction such as this one may become overly defensive at times. Distinctions like these are typically vulnerable to hard cases, where the distinction is difficult to draw at all, or where particular cases falling on either side of the line do not look all that different. There are numerous instances where lines are drawn that make useful, morally defensible distinctions for which good reasons can be given, but that remain vulnerable to certain hard cases. An example is the prohibition against performance-enhancing drugs in sport. It too relies on the therapy-enhancement distinction, but for a different purpose—determining what substances athletes are permitted to take. Efforts have been made to obliterate the distinction with hard cases, but so far they have not succeeded. Most people, including most athletes, understand that there is a difference between using a drug to treat an illness, like insulin for diabetes, and using a drug to gain a competitive advantage. They also believe the distinction is useful in practice for deciding what athletes may and may not use. There is controversy aplenty over drug-testing in sports, but the bulk of the controversy is over how to make such a testing program effective, not over the usefulness or moral legitimacy of the distinction between therapy and enhancement.

Conclusion

Whether the fruits of the Human Genome Project are sweet or bitter depends largely on how successful we are in dealing with the ethical issues it raises. There will be difficult issues of justice to be resolved, and there will be temptations to use genome-inspired technologies for enhancement rather than therapy. Our best strategy at this time is to continue to strive for justice in access to health care, and to resist efforts to obliterate the distinction between therapy and enhancement.

Notes

1. Bosk, Charles, *All God's Mistakes: Genetic Counseling in a Pediatric Hospital* (Chicago: University of Chicago Press, 1992).
2. Asch's chapter in this volume makes a similar point.
3. Mehlman, chapter 6, this volume.

Twelve

The Genetic Factor in Health Care Reform
Framing the Policy Debate

Mark A. Rothstein

A frequently used metaphor for the Human Genome Project is the prism, which refracts seemingly clear light into a spectrum of genetic variability (Boyle, 1992; Duster, 1990). The ethical, legal, and social implications of the Human Genome Project, however, also may be represented by a different optic metaphor—the convex lens of a magnifying glass, which concentrates an intense beam of light on a particular spot. When the focus is on the public and private framework for allocating access to health care, the effect of the Human Genome Project may be to intensify the scrutiny of an already precarious system and to increase the pressure to establish or reconfigure broad public policies.

Modern medical science has been driven by a technological imperative largely unquestioned since the Enlightenment. More knowledge was always good. Even if there were no immediate benefits to humankind, advances in scientific knowledge were a good per se. The Human Genome Project, perhaps more than any other biomedical undertaking, raises profound issues of whether all new information is good, whether some medical information is not empowering but disempowering, whether society has the inclination or ability to afford equal access to a powerful new technology, and whether the legal system can deal effectively with the potential for discrimination, limits on autonomy, and political divisiveness of genetic information.

Many of these difficult issues have been addressed in the thought-provoking chapters that the editors have had the privilege of assembling in this volume. In particular, the contributions of Professors Mehlman, Bobinski, Stone, and Asch help to point the way for the establishment of the public policy initiatives suggested at the end of this chapter.

Problems Arising from
Public Finance of Health Care

Maxwell J. Mehlman's chapter, "Access to the Genome and Federal Entitlement Programs," considers the ways in which expensive new genetic technology may be allocated or rationed directly or indirectly under federal and federal/state entitlement programs. He notes that genetic services may be excluded altogether as either "experimental" or as "not essential" (in an Oregon-style ranking of essential health care priorities) (Thomas, 1993). Means testing is another method that could be used to exclude from eligibility individuals above a certain income level. In addition, indirect limits could be placed on availability by simply failing to take affirmative measures to cure existing shortages of genetic services providers in certain geographic areas or by centralizing genetic treatment centers.

It is almost impossible to assess the ultimate outcome of public policies in an area such as prenatal genetic testing. Pressures to include an ever-increasing number of prenatal tests come from commercial interests of test developers and (currently) procedure-based reimbursement of providers. Patient demand for the latest medical developments and physician concern with avoiding possible malpractice liability also encourage more prenatal genetic testing (Andrews, 1992).

Yet, there also may be social pressures against providing genetic services at all, or at least publicly funding them, particularly when a likely effect of increasing the number of prenatal genetic tests is an increase in the number of abortions. Among other reasons why quality genetic services may lag behind demand is the lack of adequately trained genetic counselors and the inability of other medical specialties to keep pace with developments in genetics (Institute of Medicine, 1993).

Mehlman goes on to observe that if federal entitlement programs deny genetic services available on the open market, there will be a disparity between rich and poor in both alleviating genetic disease and, perhaps at some point in the future, gaining access to genetic enhancement. This allocative issue raises profound concerns about distributive justice. For example, if access to prenatal genetic testing and abortion were limited to affluent people, then poor people would bear a disproportionate burden of genetic disease. What would be the social consequences?

Although the Human Genome Project raises the magnitude of the cost containment issue, the basic issue is not unique. In his 1974 book, *The Ethics of Genetic Control*, Joseph Fletcher provides the following illustration: "In a southern university hospital recently a young man's hemophilia was reckoned to have cost his family, the hospital, and the public pocket a total of one million dollars by the time he decided to *marry and have children of his own*" (Fletcher, 1974).

It is possible that the prospect or reality of genetic disease frequencies skewed by income level (and therefore by race and ethnicity as well) could increase the public's willingness to use limited health care dollars to provide genetic testing instead of other medical services. On the other hand, it is perhaps more likely that additional allocations for genetic testing would not be made and that genetic diseases would become increasingly stigmatized as diseases of the poor. This consequence might actually lead to a decrease in funding for research and treatment. To some extent, this phenomenon can be seen in the public response to substance abuse. If illicit substance abuse is viewed as a problem of the suburbs, the solution is frequently education and treatment. If it is viewed as a problem of the inner cities, the answer is frequently more law enforcement.

Like many other issues related to the Human Genome Project, however, there always seems to be an alternative scenario. Although I believe it is a much less likely scenario, it could be argued that if wealthy people have access to future gene therapy and other treatment and supportive services for affected children and adults, then they will be less likely to abort a fetus with a genetic disorder. Poor people, to the extent they have access to prenatal genetic testing, would not be able to afford any alternative to abortion. Therefore, even though poor people would have less autonomy and fewer choices, they would not bear a disproportionate burden of genetic disease.

Lurking only slightly below the surface of any discussion of social policies affecting the distribution of genetic disease is the specter of eugenics. The term "eugenics" was coined in 1883 by Francis Galton to refer to the science of improving the human race through selective marriage (Smith, 1993). It comes from the Greek, meaning "good birth" (Horgan, 1993). This "positive" eugenics quickly gave way to a more sinister form of "improving the race." By sterilizing individuals with less desirable traits, such as feeble-mindedness, mental retardation, "pauperism," criminality, and epilepsy, eugenicists claimed that the population stock also could be improved—and more quickly and dramatically (Beckwith, 1993). Negative eugenics developed in the United States during the 1920s, and tens of thousands of people were sterilized. Sadly, it was American sterilization laws that inspired the Nazis who, in addition to other even more heinous crimes against humanity, sterilized over two million people between 1933 and 1945 (Kevles, 1985, Proctor, 1988).

Is it possible that the Human Genome Project could lead to a rebirth of negative eugenics, as some commentators have argued (Duster, 1990)? If there are pressures to avoid the birth of children with certain genetic disorders, in my view it will almost certainly be caused by concerns about health care cost containment.

The following incident, which arose at the Baylor College of Medicine in Houston, already has been widely reported (Billings et al., 1992). A couple from Louisiana at risk for cystic fibrosis (CF) requested prenatal genetic testing at Baylor through their Louisiana health maintenance organization (HMO). When the test was positive, the couple decided not to terminate the pregnancy. The HMO then told them that, having paid for the genetic testing, if the woman did not have an abortion, then the child's medical condition would be considered a preexisting condition not covered by the HMO. Eventually, the HMO was persuaded to change its mind and it agreed to cover the child. But, what eugenic/cost-containment pressures might exist not only to abort an affected fetus, but to prevent conception when there is a risk of a child being born with an expensive medical condition?

The HMO's reaction to the CF test seems particularly callous and unreasonable for several reasons. The illness itself is increasingly treatable and life expectancy for someone born today with CF is approximately 30 years of age, even if there were no new medical advances. Moreover, it is not clear what the couple's view of abortion was before the test was performed. There may be some medical and social benefits in learning in advance that a particular child will be born with CF. Yet, CF testing on a population-wide basis would not be a cost-effective use of medical resources unless a substantial percentage of the women with positive tests decided to terminate their pregnancies (Wilfond and Fost, 1990; Office of Technology Assessment, 1992).

Like many difficult bioethics questions, decision making after prenatal genetic testing may be easier to resolve in the abstract than in real life. It is hard to predict how any individual will react until actually confronted with the test results. Binding people to irrevocable choices in such weighty matters seems unjust. Thus, it should be irrelevant in the CF case whether the couple had not decided what to do if the test were positive or if they had decided to have an abortion and changed their minds. Furthermore, it would be extremely problematic if the couple's selection of the HMO (assuming they knew the HMO's policy on CF) should act as a waiver of their right to health care for their child (Havighurst, 1992).

The relative ease of deciding the equities of the CF example should not obscure the fact that increasingly difficult cases are inevitable. For example, suppose that a woman's first child is born with osteogenesis imperfecta, Niemann-Pick disease, or Canavan disease. Assume further that the child lives for an agonizing year and costs $500,000 or $1 million to treat. If the same woman later becomes pregnant with another affected fetus, is it reasonable for society to incur another million dollars in health care costs when treatment is largely futile and the prognosis is still so poor?

If there is to be some mechanism in place that will deny additional treatment to the child or discourage the birth of the child in the first instance, what is the rationale? Is it that the money could be better spent? That the prognosis is so poor? Or is it that the mother was irresponsible in permitting herself to have another affected child under the circumstances? Any rationale that leads to such a major limitation on the fundamental right to procreate and the right to health care must be carefully grounded (Robertson, 1990). And merely accepting the premise that cost containment may justify incursions into reproductive autonomy still does not address the issue of at what stage (preconception, prenatal, postnatal) it would be reasonable to sanction cost-conscious intervention.

From the foregoing discussion, it is obvious that once negative eugenics for cost containment purposes is considered acceptable at all, it will be extremely difficult to draw lines and the societal and psychological burdens of drawing the lines will be excruciating.

The Genome Project and Reproductive Autonomy

In Mary Anne Bobinski's chapter, "Genetics and Reproductive Decision Making," Bobinski begins by exploring the range of increasingly difficult choices facing individuals at various stages of reproduction. She considers these issues as complicating intimate personal decisions imposed by a more sophisticated understanding of genetics. The burden of an ever-expanding knowledge base also interferes with patient-professional relationships in genetics and, as she observes, adds "another layer of complexity to the genetic counseling process."

Bobinski recognizes that the pressures felt by women in reproductive decision making, for the foreseeable future, will center around the decision whether to abort a child with a genetic disorder (Clayton, 1992). For very severe disorders (e.g., anencephaly) on one extreme as well as minor conditions (e.g., polydactyly) on the other, the decision for many women may be relatively easy. Most cases, however, are likely to fall within the two extremes and therefore are likely to be much more difficult. For example, the case may involve speculation about whether a serious, late-onset disorder that is largely untreatable today (e.g., amyotrophic lateral sclerosis) will be treatable by the time the individual would become symptomatic. This would be a difficult assessment even for an expert medical geneticist and therefore is a virtually impossible task for a layperson with the added psychological pressures of parenthood. As Barbara Katz Rothman has written, "You are asking [women] to evaluate what kind of life is worth living" (Rothman, 1986).

Thus far I have observed that the issue of when it is appropriate for society to intervene to avoid the birth of a child with a genetic disorder will depend on medical, economic, political, social, and psychological factors involving the affected individual and his or her parents. There are other third parties, however, with a great interest in these issues. For example, some disability-rights advocates are concerned about societal programs to avoid the birth of individuals with disabilities. They argue, in effect, that efforts to avoid the birth of children with disorders such as spina bifida, Down's syndrome, and cerebral palsy are tantamount to a societal declaration that individuals already affected with these disorders have less intrinsic worth and are less valuable members of society. Thus, they argue that respect for human dignity, human biodiversity, and (in some cases) for religious reasons, prenatal genetic testing should not be performed because it leads to eugenic abortions.

This position, which can lead to outright opposition to the Human Genome Project, overlooks both the principle of autonomy and the project's vast potential to alleviate human suffering. Knowledge of the process by which genes code for the development of proteins and other gene products and how these products affect disease will have major effects on somatic cell gene therapy as well as more traditional pharmaceutical interventions. The availability of treatment could well lead to a decrease in the demand for abortion for a wide range of genetic disorders. Genetic research is not necessarily inconsistent with increased supportive services for already affected individuals nor with a greater tolerance for phenotypical diversity.

Bobinski goes on to analyze the range of potential governmental responses at the legislative and judicial levels. She paints the picture of federal and state governments that might mandate (to reduce genetic disease) or prohibit (because of cost considerations or to discourage abortion) genetic testing. Governments might attempt to prevent procreation (through sterilization) or restrict abortions. They might attempt to regulate gene therapy or genetic engineering. Astonishingly, the state and federal governments could attempt to implement several inconsistent policies simultaneously.

After considering the constitutionality of each of the possible governmental activities, Bobinski recognizes that the wisest course for the government is to leave control of procreation to the parents. In the short run, at least, that may be easier said than done, considering the depth of emotion underlying reproduction. Government abstinence would represent more than an endorsement of autonomy. It would reflect a degree of tolerance often lacking in today's public discourse. After all, the right to control one's own reproduction is a right to bring about consequences that invariably run counter to the values of some segment of society.

Private Health Insurance Reform

In the United States today, 85 to 90 percent of health insurance is purchased through group health plans, with about three-fourths of the groups based on employment. In small groups, as with individual policies, there is some individual medical underwriting. For large groups, however, there is little individual medical underwriting, although there may be "risk finder" or "gatekeeper" questions on the master insurance application, which seek to determine the experience of the group (Stone, 1993).

Numerous books and articles have been written about the possible use of genetic screening in health insurance and the threat that individuals most in need of health insurance will be denied coverage (Rothstein, 1993). There is widespread agreement, including among many health insurers, that denying health insurance on the basis of a predictive genetic test is socially unacceptable. Moreover, once one health insurance company undertakes such a policy, the insurance market will become further segmented. Then there will be increased pressure on other insurers also to use genetic test results. Before long, it will be impossible to spread risks effectively (Task Force, 1993).

Deborah A. Stone's chapter, "The Implications of the Human Genome Project for Access to Health Insurance," takes up the often-debated issue of what the effect of the new genetics will be on the health insurance industry. In her view, compared with other forms of medical information, the difference is in degree rather than in kind. "Genetic information may hold a special fascination in our collective imagination, but its use in and impact on health insurance will be only a change in degree from the status quo, not a fundamental transformation." Moreover, as Stone observes, as research focuses less on monogenic disorders and more on common, multifactorial disorders, it will be increasingly difficult to define what is a "genetic" disease or even a "genetic" test. Stone correctly notes that there are many proposed answers, but most of them address the wrong question. The problem is more fundamental than the effect of genetic information on the health insurance system; it is the viability and fairness of the system itself.

There is a tendency to assume that genetic screening and genetic discrimination in health insurance are not realistic possibilities for the future, but mere conjecture based on the temporary anomaly of our current health care system. After all, the American health care system is likely to undergo sweeping changes in the coming years. Current health insurance practices, such as using predictive screening, preexisting condition clauses, exclusion waivers, risk underwriting, experience rating, cancellation clauses, and maximum premium increases are likely to be unlawful even without a comprehensive new health care system. Thus, in the future there would be no value to genetic screening that was not clinically indicated because the results could not be used by insurers or providers to restrict access to health care. Consequently, a myriad of problems will be eliminated in one fell swoop by a new health care system—from privacy and confidentiality to stigmatization and injustice.

There is only one problem with this hypothesis: it is unlikely to comport with reality. A new American health care system that would provide a comprehensive package of benefits to every citizen is politically dubious and it would be extremely expensive. It would need to provide meaningful health care access not only to the estimated 37 million uninsured Americans, but it would also need to provide care for at least an equal number of underinsured people as well as the "insured but medically underserved." Consequently, any universal access health care plan is unlikely to cover the full range of medical services, such as mental health, substance abuse treatment, long-term care, and various elective surgeries and diagnostic procedures. Under a limited public health care system, there still would be a need for private health insurance companies to offer the supplemental coverage plans that virtually all people who could afford them will want to purchase.

If it is assumed that genetic screening by health insurance companies violates public policy, where the effect is to deny individuals access to basic and essential health services, are the public policy issues the same when the insurance policy is nonessential and supplemental? The answer is far from clear. It would depend upon the predictive value of the genetic tests, the assurances of confidentiality, and other factors. Most importantly, however, it would depend on what health care coverage was included in the basic package. If an individual wants to purchase deluxe coverage to obtain cosmetic surgery, with private duty nurses and a private hospital suite, an argument could be made that an insurer offering such coverage should have a right to require whatever medical information it wants. On the other hand, if the supplemental coverage is needed to, for example, provide basic mental health services, then genetic screening to determine insurance eligibility would violate public policy.

Although the United States leads the world in per capita health care costs, substantial annual increases in health care costs are not unique to the United States. Many of the increased costs around the world have been dictated by new, expensive medical technologies. Indeed, it has been estimated that 50 percent of the health care cost increase in the United States in 1992 was caused by new technology. These universal cost pressures and political realities make it quite likely that within 10 years there will be a convergence of many of the various health care systems in the industrialized nations. Specifically, the private sector will play a greater role in other parts of the world, such as Western Europe. Accordingly, it is probable that the typical health care system will feature a limited, austere, guaranteed medical benefits package, with private, supplemental coverage insurance policies common. For example, in Australia 40 percent of the population already purchases private health insurance to supplement the government's "Medicare" system (McIlwaine, 1993).

The debate and the ensuing questions engendered by the Human Genome Project in the United States are destined to be played out in many lands. What package of government-mandated or government-provided health benefits should be available unconditionally? What personal medical information do individuals have a right to keep private? What individual medical information do health insurers have a legitimate right to know to avoid adverse selection for nonessential medical insurance? The inevitability of answering these questions makes it apparent that the issue of genetic information and health insurance is neither premature nor likely to be mooted by any type of public or private health care reform.

The Role of Employers

It is not clear what role employers will play in the future American health care system, although it is probably unrealistic to assume that they will play no role. Thus, if employers maintain a financial stake in employee health insurance, the question must be asked whether changes in health insurance will simply shift the incentive to discriminate from the insurer to the employer. For example, under a system in which the additional costs of each health benefits claim are borne directly (through self-insurance) or indirectly (through experience rating) by employers, they have tremendous incentives to discriminate against actual or perceived high-cost users of health benefits (Rothstein, 1989). The ability to use genetic technologies in the predictive screening process increases the societal risks of such a system. Unfortunately, it is not clear whether current antidiscrimination laws, principally the Americans with Disabilities Act, will protect against genetic-based discrimination (Rothstein, 1992).

In her chapter, "Genetics and Employment: More Disability Discrimination," Adrienne Asch writes of the profound misfit between the objectives of a just health care system and the risk aversion of employers. By 1991, 65 percent of all employers were self-insured and 82 percent of large employers (with 5,000 or more employees) were self-insured (A. Foster Higgins, 1992). Self-insured employers are exempt from state health insurance regulation, including mandated health benefits laws and high-risk insurance pools. Yet, the pressures to limit future health claims are felt just as acutely by self-insured employers as commercial insurers. In addition, the effects of defensive measures by employers are even more devastating, because employers may be tempted to exclude high-cost users (regardless of legal considerations), and to the extent permitted, to restrict the range of health benefits or eliminate health benefits altogether.

Politically, we have recently witnessed the public's aversion to sweeping, government-imposed changes to the health care system. Even the most sweeping proposals, however, would have maintained an important role for employers. The Health Security Act proposed by the Clinton administration would have permitted employers with 5,000 or more employees to opt out of proposed health care alliances. Other bills set the opt-out level at 100. Because self-insured employers pay health care bills directly rather than purchasing insurance from an insurance company, the employer bears the risk entirely. Therefore, any self-insured employer has a tremendous financial incentive to exclude from employment perceived high-cost users of health care. The smaller the employer, the less ability it has to spread risks over a large group of workers and to absorb a large loss. Consequently, a relatively smaller self-insured company would be under tremendous pressure to have a below-average loss experience and, notwithstanding legal proscriptions, to exclude certain individuals from employment.

The prospect of continued or even expanded self-insurance raises the possibility that health-based discrimination will not be eliminated, but merely shifted from insurers to employers. If employers, including self-insured employers, are to have a role in financing the new health care system, the employer role should be limited to paying a flat, per capita assessment in the form of a tax or premium contribution. This would remove the incentive to obtain predictive medical information and to use the information to modify health benefits or to discriminate in employment opportunities.

In her chapter, Asch makes two other points that deserve further comment. She joins Deborah Stone in the view that it is futile to try to differentiate between genetic and nongenetic illness. Some obvious definitional problems are raised by tests that measure gene products or effects, by multifactorial disorders, and by constantly changing scientific understanding. Even if such distinctions could be drawn, they would still be meaningless. The basic issues of enhancing health and dignity are the same. It is only because of inappropriate legal constraints that the genetic/nongenetic issue exists at all. In a similar vein, Asch reminds us that the denial of employment opportunities—long suffered by people with disabilities—often brings with it devastating psychosocial consequences.

Toward a Policy and Legislative Agenda

Ever since the Ethical, Legal, and Social Implications (ELSI) program of the Human Genome Project got under way, a variety of fascinating conferences, workshops, meetings, and academic writings have pondered the future social consequences of the Human Genome Project. We may still have the luxury of further pondering and reflecting in some areas, but with regard to access to health care, it is time to translate the social concerns expressed in this book and elsewhere into meaningful, appropriate action.

First, in devising national health strategy the importance of emerging genetic technologies must be recognized. This means not just a commitment to fund genome research, but to increase substantially public and professional education in genetics. It means that essential, appropriate genetic services must be covered by reimbursement systems. For example, while population screening for carriers of recessive disorders such as CF need not be funded where medically unindicated, presymptomatic testing of people at risk for Huntington's disease should be made available. Furthermore, affirmative steps must be taken to remove the nonfinancial barriers to access to genetic services, such as geographical isolation, lack of transportation, language barriers, and cultural barriers.

We also need to ensure an adequate supply of genetic services providers. Currently, fewer than one-third of all physicians are engaged in primary care. In the newly-emerging health care system, one-half of all physicians will be in primary care. Primary care physicians and their nurses will be responsible for a substantial amount of genetic counseling and referrals. This reality underscores the need for additional emphasis on genetics in medical and nursing schools as well as in continuing education programs.

Second, autonomous reproductive decision making must be a primary public health goal. To value autonomy is to value the ability of individuals to make decisions with which the majority or those in positions of power sometimes disagree. In the area of prenatal genetic testing, our policy must attempt to strike a balance between ensuring the freedom of choice to terminate a pregnancy while resisting negative eugenic pressures encouraging abortion that could stem from efforts to control health care costs. The result may well be the abortion of some fetuses with congenital anomalies that most people would consider minor, as well as the birth of some children with profound or lethal genetic conditions where most people would terminate the pregnancy. Yet, I would argue that the societal costs at the margins caused by a relatively few "unpopular" or "inappropriate" decisions at either end of the continuum will be far less than the societal costs that would come with the loss of essential reproductive freedoms.

An argument could be made that many abortions are currently performed for economic reasons—the mother or family cannot support the child. Therefore, it could be asserted that it is not immoral for society to require the abortion of a child that the government cannot afford to treat. Nevertheless, there is a significant difference between an individual's decision to terminate a pregnancy for whatever reason and governmental coercion to do so.

Third, encounters with the medical-genetic establishment will become increasingly complicated. It is too late in the process to assume that detailed educational programs and genetic counseling at the clinical stage will be sufficient to assist individuals in making decisions with which they are comfortable. We simply do not have enough genetic counselors or other comparably trained health care providers to explain complex genetic conditions and mathematical probabilities to individuals with no background at all in genetics. Human genetics education must be stressed in the public schools and in other appropriate forums, so that health care consumers are better prepared to deal with the complexities of emerging technologies (Institute of Medicine, 1993).

Fourth, the use of genetic testing or genetic information by health insurance companies should be illegal unless and until every citizen is entitled to a basic health benefits package that assures adequate health care for a comprehensive range of conditions. If such a package is in place and individuals want to purchase deluxe, premium health insurance coverage, insurers should be permitted to require the use of any form of predictive medical test for medical underwriting so long as there is a sound actuarial basis for doing so, the decision making process is fair, and strict standards of confidentiality are maintained. State legislation restricting the use of genetic tests or genetic information in health insurance is a largely futile gesture in the absence of comprehensive health care reform.

Fifth, discrimination in employment on the basis of a genotype that affects a major life activity or is regarded as doing so should be illegal, either through amendment of the Americans with Disabilities Act (ADA) or interpretation of the statute by the Equal Employment Opportunity Commission (EEOC) or the courts. An individual with an atypical genotype should be considered an individual with a disability for purposes of the ADA. Genetic predisposition to illness should be considered the same as any other increased medical risk. Although a 1995 interpretation by the EEOC provides that genetic predisposition to disease is a disability under the ADA, this issue has not yet been decided by the courts. Moreover, this interpretation does not afford coverage to unaffected carriers of recessive and x-linked disorders who may be subject to discrimination by employers concerned about possible health care costs of dependents.

Another employment issue to be resolved concerns whether employers may perform genetic tests on individuals who have been made a conditional offer of employment. The text of the ADA does not resolve the issue and EEOC has taken the position that post-offer medical examinations are not limited by the ADA. Therefore, these examinations may delve into any medical subjects, even if they have no bearing on the job. Although the law in one state, Minnesota, already bans such needlessly intrusive inquiries, the ADA does not. Accordingly, under the ADA all medical examinations mandated by employers should be limited to the assessment of the individual's ability to perform specific job-related functions. Moreover, employers seeking access to employee medical records also should be limited only to job-related medical information. Thus, employers should not be permitted to require the signing of blanket releases of all medical records in the possession of an individual's private physician.

Sixth, genetic information must be strictly limited to health care providers. There are a number of potential uses of genetic information beyond insurance and employment. For example, an individual's genotype could be used in education, finance, government benefits and services, and other areas (Alper and Natowicz, 1993). Any person or entity with a financial interest in learning the likely future health status of an individual might want to see that individual's genetic profile. New microcomputer technology, including credit card–sized optical memory cards, will facilitate these compelled disclosures (Gostin et al., 1993; Office of Technology Assessment, 1993; Rothstein, 1993a). New laws are needed to prohibit the use of genetic information except in health care, forensics, and other narrowly tailored situations. We must ensure that genetic information does not become a commodity that is widely available on the market.

Conclusion

Although sweeping health care reform is unlikely in the United States for the foreseeable future, this does not mean that we have the luxury to overlook the effects of new discoveries in genetics on our health care system or society. Our public health and health finance policies must respect the autonomy, privacy, confidentiality, diversity, and informed decision making of all Americans. It is not too soon to begin incorporating the public policies outlined above into concrete legislative and health care initiatives.

References

A. Foster Higgins & Co., Foster Higgins Health Care Benefits Survey, 1991 (1992).

Alper, Joseph S., and Natowicz, Marvin R., "Genetic Discrimination and the Public Entities and Public Accommodations Titles of the Americans with Disabilities Act," American Journal of Human Genetics, 53:26 (1993).

Andrews, Lori B., "Torts and the Double Helix: Malpractice Liability for Failure to Warn of Genetic Risks," Houston Law Review, 29:149 (1992).

Beckwith, Jon, "A Historical View of Social Responsibility in Genetics," BioScience, 43:327 (1993).

Billings, Paul, et al., "Discrimination as a Consequence of Genetic Testing," American Journal of Human Genetics, 50:476 (1992).

Boyle, Philip J., "Genetic Grammar: 'Health,' 'Illness,' and the Human

Genome Project," Special Supplement, Hastings Center Report, vol. 22, no. 4, at S1 (1992).

Clayton, Ellen Wright, "Screening and Treatment of Newborns," Houston Law Review, 29:85 (1992).

Duster, Troy, *Backdoor to Eugenics* (1990).

Fletcher, Joseph, *The Ethics of Genetic Control* (1974).

Gostin, Lawrence O., "Privacy and Security of Personal Information in a New Health Care System," JAMA, 270:2487 (1993).

Havighurst, Clark C., "Prospective Self-Denial: Can Consumers Contract Today to Accept Health Care Rationing Tomorrow?," University of Pennsylvania Law Review, 140:1755 (1992).

Horgan, John, "Eugenics Revisited," *Scientific America*, June 1993, 122.

Institute of Medicine, National Academy of Sciences, "Assessing Genetic Risks: Implications for Health and Social Policy" (1993).

Kevles, Daniel J., *In the Name of Eugenics* (1985).

McIlwaine, Kate, "Australia: Dissatisfaction Despite Low Inflation," Business Insurance, March 26, 1993, 45.

Office of Technology Assessment, U.S. Congress, "Cystic Fibrosis and DNA Tests: Implications of Carrier Screening" (1992).

Office of Technology Assessment, U.S. Congress, "Protecting Privacy in Computerized Medical Information" (1993).

Proctor, Robert, *Racial Hygiene: Medicine under the Nazis* (1988).

Robertson, John A., "Procreative Liberty and Human Genetics," Emory Law Journal 39:697 (1990).

Rothman, Barbara Katz, *The Tentative Pregnancy* (1986).

Rothstein, Mark A., "Genetic Discrimination in Employment and the Americans with Disabilities Act," Houston Law Review, 29:23 (1992).

Rothstein, Mark A., "Genetics, Insurance, and the Ethics of Genetic Counseling," in *Molecular Genetic Medicine*, vol. 3, T. Friedmann, ed. (1993).

Rothstein, Mark A., "Toward a Patient-Centered View of Health Care Reform," Journal of American Health Policy, Sept.–Oct., 1993 (1993a).

Rothstein, Mark A., *Medical Screening and the Employee Health Cost Crisis* (1989).

Smith, J. David, *The Eugenic Assault on America* (1993).

Stone, Deborah A., "The Struggle for the Soul of Health Insurance," Journal of Health Politics, Policy & Law, 18:287 (1993).

Task Force on Genetic Information and Insurance, NIH/DOE Working Group on Ethical, Legal, and Social Implications of Human Genome Research, Genetic Information and Health Insurance (1993).

Thomas, W. John, "The Oregon Medicaid Proposal: Ethical Paralysis, Tragic Democracy, and the Fate of a Utilitarian Health Care Program," Oregon Law Review, 72:47 (1993).

Wilfond, Benjamin S., and Fost, Norman, "The Cystic Fibrosis Gene: Medical and Social Implications for Heterozygote Detection," JAMA, 263:2777 (1990).

Contributors

W. French Anderson, M.D., was formerly Chief, Molecular Hematology Branch for the National Institutes of Health at Bethesda, Maryland, and is presently Professor of Biochemistry and Pediatrics at the University of Southern California School of Medicine in Los Angeles.

Adrienne Asch, Ph.D., ACSW, CSW, is Henry R. Luce Professor in Biology, Ethics, and the Politics of Human Reproduction at Wellesley College, and was a member of the Hillary Rodham Clinton Health Care Task Force, Bioethics Working Group. She received her Ph.D. in Social Psychology from Columbia University, and was Associate in Social Science and Policy at the New Jersey Bioethics Commission. Dr. Asch has published in the areas of ethical issues in genetics, reproductive technology, abortion, and disability.

Mary Anne Bobinski is Associate Professor at the University of Houston Law Center where she is also the Associate Director for J.D. Programs of the Health Law and Policy Institute. She received her J.D. from the State University of New York at Buffalo and her LL.M. from Harvard Law School. Professor Bobinski writes and speaks on reproductive health law issues, HIV-related legal issues, and the legal implications of health care finance and reform.

Norman Daniels is Goldthwaite Professor and former Chair of the Philosophy Department and Professor of Medical Ethics, Tufts Medical School. He received his doctorate from Harvard University. Dr. Daniels is a Fellow of the Hastings Center, has served as a member of the Ethics

Working Group of the Clinton White House Health Care Task Force, and is currently a member of the Public Health Service Expert Panel on Cost Effectiveness and Clinical Preventive Medicine. His many publications include *Just Health Care, Am I My Parents' Keeper? An Essay on Justice between the Young and the Old, Seeking Fair Treatment: From the AIDS Epidemic to National Health Care Reform, Justice and Justification: Reflective Equilibrium in Theory and Practice* (forthcoming), and (with Donald Light and Ronald Caplan) *Benchmarks of Fairness for Health Care Reform*, which is also forthcoming.

Albert R. Jonsen, Ph.D., is Professor and Chair, Department of Medical History and Ethics, University of Washington School of Medicine. He received his doctorate from the Department of Religious Studies at Yale University. He has served as Chief of the Division of Medical Ethics at the School of Medicine, University of California, San Francisco, and was President of the University of San Francisco, where he taught in the departments of Philosophy and Theology. Dr. Jonsen is currently Chair of the newly established National Advisory Board on Ethics in Reproduction (NABER). Among the honors he has received are the McGovern Award of the American Osler Society, the Annual Award of the Society for Health and Human Values, and the Davies Award of the American College of Physicians. His publications include *The New Medicine and the Old Ethics* and *The Abuse of Casuistry: A History of Moral Reasoning*.

Maxwell J. Mehlman, J.D., is Professor of Law and Director of the Law-Medicine Center, Case Western Reserve University School of Law. He received his J.D. from Yale Law School and holds two bachelor's degrees, one from Reed College and one from Oxford University, which he attended as a Rhodes Scholar. Prior to joining the faculty at CWRU, Professor Mehlman practiced law with Arnold & Porter in Washington, D.C., where he specialized in federal regulation of medical technology. Professor Mehlman writes and lectures on a number of issues in law and medicine, including the just allocation of scarce resources, the Human Genome Project, medical malpractice reform, and the role of the health professional under the common law.

Robert F. Murray, Jr., M.D., is Chief of the Division of Medical Genetics in the Department of Pediatrics and Child Health, and Professor of Pediatrics, Medicine, and Genetics. He is also Chair of the Graduate Department of Genetics and Human Genetics at Howard University.

Dr. Murray is an active member of the Institute of Medicine of the National Academy of Sciences, a fellow and member of the Board of Directors of the Hastings Center on Bioethics, and a Fellow of the American Association for the Advancement of Science. He has served on special committees at the National Institutes of Health such as the Recombinant DNA Advisory Committee (RAC) and the Human Gene Therapy Subcommittee of the RAC and the recently established Working Group on Ethics, Law and Social Issues of the National Center for Human Genome Research. Dr. Murray is co-author with Dr. James Bowman of *Genetic Variation and Disorders in Peoples of African Origin.*

Thomas H. Murray, Ph.D., is Professor and Director of the Center for Biomedical Ethics at Case Western Reserve University. A founding member of the Ethical, Legal, and Social Issues Working Group for the Human Genome Project in the United States, Professor Murray serves on its international counterpart in HUGO—The Human Genome Organization. He also chaired the Task Force on Genetic Information and Insurance. His interest in the ethics of enhancement is reinforced by ten years of work with the United States Olympic Committee's efforts to deal with performance-enhancing drugs in sports.

Herbert Nickens, M.D., M.A., is the first Vice President and Director of the Division of Community and Minority Programs at the Association of American Medical Colleges in Washington, D.C. Before his current position, Dr. Nickens was the first Director of the Office of Minority Health, U.S. Department of Health and Human Services. He has also held the positions of Director, Office of Policy, Planning, and Analysis of the National Institute on Aging, and Deputy Chief, Center on Aging, National Institutes of Mental Health. Dr. Nickens has written numerous articles, lectured frequently on geriatrics, minority health, and AIDS, and has made a number of appearances on radio and television programs. He is board certified by the American Board of Psychiatry and Neurology. He also received the History of Medicine Prize from the University of Pennsylvania in 1973, and in 1978 the Kenneth Appel Award from the Philadelphia County Medical Society, and the Laughlin Prize from the National Psychiatric Endowment Fund.

William J. Polvino, M.D., was formerly a Fellow at the Molecular Hematology Branch for the National Institutes of Health at Bethesda, Maryland, and is presently Associate Director, Clinical Pharmacology at Merck Research Laboratories in Rahway, New Jersey.

Vincent M. Riccardi, M.D., is founder and Director of the Neurofibromatosis Institute in La Crescenta, California, is founder of the Colorado-Wyoming Regional Genetic Counseling Program, and also of the journal *Neurofibromatosis*. He is board-certified in Internal Medicine, Clinical Genetics and Clinical Cytogenetics, and is a Fellow of the American College of Physicians, the American Association for the Advancement of Science, and the American College of Medical Genetics. Dr. Riccardi has published extensively in the areas of neurofibromatosis and other topics in human genetics, including *Neurofibromatosis: Phenotype, Natural History, and Pathogenesis*. In the field of human genetics, Dr. Riccardi has made several contributions, including delineation of the trisomy 8 syndrome; discovery of the deletion in the short arm of chromosome 11 and eventually the WT1 gene that accounts for some patients having the childhood cancer, Wilms Tumor; discovery of the deletion in the long arm of chromosome 15 accounting for many cases of the Prader-Willi syndrome; and research on the chromosomal mechanism to explain Rett syndrome. His research in neurofibromatosis has contributed substantially to the understanding of the natural history and molecular genetics of this disorder.

Mark A. Rothstein, J.D., is Hugh Roy and Lillie Cranz Cullen Distinguished Professor of Law and Director of the Health Law and Policy Institute at the University of Houston. He received a B.A. from the University of Pittsburgh and a J.D. from Georgetown University. Professor Rothstein was a member of the Committee on Assessing Genetic Risks of the Institute of Medicine of the National Academy of Sciences and served as a legal consultant to the National Center for Human Genome Research of the National Institutes of Health. He has written nearly 100 articles and is the author or co-author of nine books.

Deborah A. Stone, Ph.D., holds the David R. Pokross Chair in Law and Social Policy at Brandeis University. She received a Ph.D. in political science from the Massachusetts Institute of Technology in 1976, and Bachelor of Arts, Magna Cum Laude, from the University of Michigan in 1969, with a major in Russian studies. She is the author of three books and numerous articles on social policy and politics, the Senior Editor of *The American Prospect*, and founding member of the National Academy of Social Insurance. She was a member of the Task Force on Genetic Information and Insurance of the Human Genome Project.

Index

Index

245